Principles of Psychology for Graduate Nurses

Principles of Psychology for Graduate Nurses

As per Revised INC Syllabus

PR Nalini
MSW MSc (Psychology)
PG Diploma in Guidance and Counseling
Visiting Professor
Bollineni College of Nursing, Nellore, Andhra Pradesh, India
Dileef College of Nursing, Nellore, Andhra Pradesh, India
Govt. College of Nursing, Nellore, Andhra Pradesh, India
St. Joseph's College of Nursing, Nellore, Andhra Pradesh, India
Narayana College of Physiotherapy, Nellore, Andhra Pradesh, India
Family Counseling Member (Women Police Station), Nellore, Andhra Pradesh, India

JAYPEE

JAYPEE BROTHERS MEDICAL PUBLISHERS

The Health Sciences Publisher

New Delhi | London

JAYPEE Jaypee Brothers Medical Publishers (P) Ltd

Headquarters
Jaypee Brothers Medical Publishers (P) Ltd
EMCA House, 23/23-B
Ansari Road, Daryaganj
New Delhi 110 002, India
Landline: +91-11-23272143, +91-11-23272703
+91-11-23282021, +91-11-23245672
Email: jaypee@jaypeebrothers.com

Corporate Office
Jaypee Brothers Medical Publishers (P) Ltd
4838/24, Ansari Road, Daryaganj
New Delhi 110 002, India
Phone: +91-11-43574357
Fax: +91-11-43574314
Email: jaypee@jaypeebrothers.com

Overseas Office
J.P. Medical Ltd
83 Victoria Street, London
SW1H 0HW (UK)
Phone: +44 20 3170 8910
Fax: +44 (0)20 3008 6180
Email: info@jpmedpub.com

Website: www.jaypeebrothers.com
Website: www.jaypeedigital.com

Principles of Psychology for Graduate Nurses

First Edition: **2021,** Reprint: 2024

ISBN: 978-93-90595-29-7

Printed in India at Rajkamal Electric Press, Kundli, Haryana.

Dedicated to

My parents Sri Vasili Venkata Ramanaiah and Annapurnamma,
My in-laws Pelluru Ramanaiah Naidu and Krishnavenamma,
My husband Sri Pelluru Rajendra Prasad and brothers
V Venkata Subbaiah and Dr Venkata Seshaiah

Preface

My education and my family helped me to get success in teaching profession in the subject Psychology. My students are getting good score and university ranks in my subject psychology by my teaching subject. These points inspired me to write this textbook for graduate nurses.

My family and friends encouraged me to work as a counseling psychologist in a family counseling center under the women police station in the present city. The District Legal Service Authority gave me a chance to work as a Family Welfare Committee member in the present city. The honorary services as family counseling member to women police station in compromising the majority of couples with the support of the department. My membership in one of the Ethics Committee of Medical groups helped me in writing script. All these experiences helped me in preparation for this textbook in a successful way. My regular participation in the International Psychotherapy Institution community virtual meeting also helped me in writing this script for the present scenario.

My teaching experience convinced me that a nursing student will be relieved from their anxiety by having a good textbook covering the topics from the present syllabus. It gives chance to concentrate more on the classroom lecture than noting down the points of the subject in the classroom.

The students of nursing are also suffering to refer to books due to lack of time to be spent in libraries. This book is useful to the nursing students, physiotherapy students and other allied health sciences.

I have referred many valuable books and sources on psychology while writing this text. This book attempts to meet the educational and professional needs of the students in strengthening the services of nurses towards patients and society. It also helps students in understanding and applying psychological knowledge in their professional lives. It has been written in simple form with suitable examples.

PR Nalini

Acknowledgments

Deep felt gratitude to my family members especially my elder brothers, Sri Venkata Subbaiah and Sri Venkata Seshaiah in encouragement towards my higher education. I am thankful to my mother Annapurnamma, my mother-in-law Krishnavenamma, my brothers and sister-in-laws who helped me in tackling several issues in family and society.

My special thanks to my brother Dr VVG Krishna Murthy (Retired DM and HO) who read the manuscript carefully and suggested valuable additions which helped me to publish this book in an elegant form. I am also thankful to my son and daughter who supported me in technical matters of writing script.

I am extremely thankful to Dr P Narayana, Chairman (Narayan Group of Medical Institutions), Sri P Tirapathi, Principal of Narayana College of Physiotherapy, Nellore, Andhra Pradesh, India, Sri B Krishnaiah, Chairman (KIMS), Sri Giri Naidu, CEO, Bollineni College of Nursing, Nellore, Andhra Pradesh, India, Sri Ashok, Principal, Bollineni College of Nursing, Nellore, Andhra Pradesh, India, Sri Prabhudas, Chairman, Dileef College of Nursing, Nellore, Andhra Pradesh, India, Smt S Komalamma, Principal, Govt. College of Nursing, Nellore, Andhra Pradesh, India, Sister Martha T, Principal, St Joseph's College of Nursing, Nellore, Andhra Pradesh, India.

I am grateful to all the authors of the reference books I have referred in the compilation of this text. My special thanks to my students who secured good marks and university ranks by my teaching which in turn inspired me to write this book. I am also grateful to class in-charges who cooperated in different aspects of my teaching.

Contents

CHAPTER 1

Introduction to Psychology

Learning Objectives

- History and origin of science of psychology
- Definitions and scope of psychology
- Relevance to nursing
- Methods of psychology

INTRODUCTION

The branch "Psychology" started as a branch of philosophy and continued for about 2,000 years before emerging as a science. Psychology helped to understand the mystic experiences, activities of people, and events which included their experiences of life, dreams, materialistic life, and the peculiar behavior of people in different situations.

The term psychology was first encountered in philosophical books of 16th century which was formed of two Greek words "psyche" (soul) and "logos" (doctrine). By the word "soul", it meant the principle underlying all the phenomena of mental and spiritual life, while the term "doctrine" meant a principle or position of the body of principles in a branch of knowledge.

HISTORY AND ORIGIN OF SCIENCE OF PSYCHOLOGY

Psychology as a subject emerged from philosophy which later developed as a separate science study about mental illness in a scientific way.

The first foundation of psychology as a science was laid by Greek physicians in 16th century BC from religion and philosophy. The study of psychology enables us to answer many questions in a scientific manner.

The modern ideas of mind have evolved from Greek philosophy. Among the plethora of prominent Greek philosophers who have made notable contribution to the development of psychology, Greek physician Alcmaeon in the 6th century is known to have laid the initial foundation of psychology as a science. In his concept the mind and soul are located in brain and it has the base for human intelligence.

From Socrates introduction about existence of mind and soul, which was accepted by his students (Plato, Aristotle) to the growing interest of Plato to know the role of mind in controlling human behavior, which further gave away to Dualism in Psychology supported by Aristotle's contribution of the idea of the inseparability of soul and living body (and the necessity to understand psychological processes including the activities of sense of organs which help the individual to experience his environment) to the emergence of French philosopher Rene Desecrates (1596–1650), who postulated the existence of soul as a separate entity which is

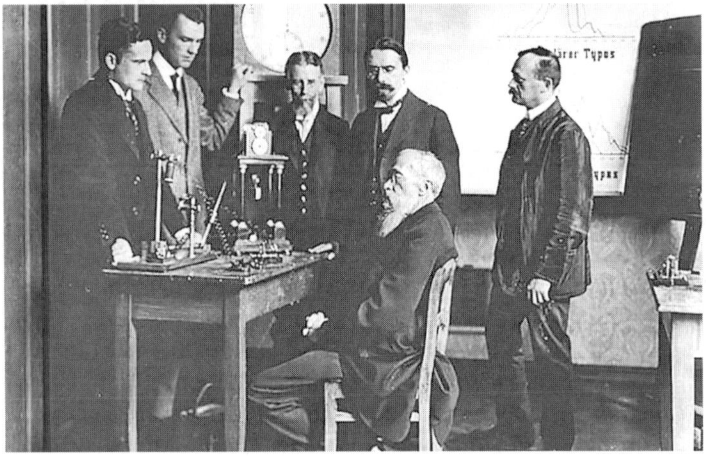

Fig. 1.1: Wilhelm Wundt (seated) with colleagues in his psychology laboratory

independent of body, psychology has witnessed a slow yet steady pace of evolving into a definite subject. With gradual development in the scientific outlook, the philosophical meaning of "psyche" changed from soul to mind because of its fading prominence.

Wilhelm James in his book "Principles of Psychology" published in 1890 defined psychology as the description and explanation of state of consciousness as such.

Later Wilhelm Wundt (1832–1920) named as the father of experimental psychology established the first Institute of Psychology in 1879 at Leipzig in Germany **(Fig. 1.1)**. Wilhelm Wundt's greatest contribution to psychology was to show that psychology could be a valid experimental science.

Psychology is defined as "The scientific study of behavior and mental processes." Later, it has developed into an independent scientific discipline in Germany and United States. Psychology is also related to the fields of physiology, neuroscience, artificial intelligence, sociology, and anthropology as well as philosophy and other components of the humanities.

In the 20th century, cognitive science got prominence to study about human mind. It is used as an important tool in psychological evolution, linguistic, computer science, behaviorism, and neurobiology. It is also helping in investigation and understanding of human mind by applying research domains such as artificial science.

Structuralism

Structuralism attempts to analyze a specific field as a complex system of interrelated parts. It proposes analyzation of human mind, thoughts that all the human activity and products of human mind including thoughts and experiences in day to day life are constructed and natural and in particular that everything has meaning because of language system in which humans operate. The main method used to discover these elementary units of mind was introspection.

Functionalism

Functionalism was initiated by William James (1842–1910), the father of American psychology. Functionalists performed experiments in learning, memory, reasoning, etc. Functionalists believed that environment has a major role toward the adjustment of the individuals.

Behaviorism

This school of thought was started by JB Watson (1878–1958) and supported by other notable psychologists including Thorndike, Pavlov, Skinner, Tolman, Hull, etc. Watson propounded that psychology was a natural science whose domain was restricted to observable events where the only objectively measurable event was organism's behavior. He insisted that psychology should be restricted to the study of the activities of people and animals—their behavior.

Gestalt Psychology

This school of thought was established in the year 1912 by three German psychologists—Max Wertheimer (1880–1941) and his colleagues Kurt Koffka (1886–1941) and Wolfgang Kohler (1887–1967).

The Gestalt believed that the mind is not made up of elements and it is possible to study mind by whole. They argued that the mind could be thought of as resulting from the whole pattern of sensory activity and the relationships are organization within pattern.

Psychoanalysis

Sigmund Freud (1856–1939) was the founding father of psychoanalysis. He developed a theory of behavior and mind on urges or drives. His theory was based on three levels of unconsciousness, sub-consciousness, and consciousness.

Major Landmarks in the Developments of Psychology

1879—Wilhelm Wundt, first psychology laboratory in Leipzig, Germany
1885—Human Ebbinghaus, study of memory process
1890—Principles of psychology published by William James
1890—James Cattell—term of mental tests
1890—Francis Galton developed intelligence studies
1892—Foundation of American Psychological Association (APA) headed by Granville Stanley Hall
1895—Alfred Binet—first laboratory of psychodiagnosis
1896—First psychological clinic at the University of Pennsylvania
1900—Sigmund Freud—psychoanalytic thought
1904—Ivan Pavlov wins Nobel Prize for work on fundamental principles of learning
1905—Alfred Binet's Intelligence Test published in France
1911—Edward Thorndike—Operant conditioning
1912—Wlliam Stern developed Intelligence Quotient Formula

$$\text{Intelligence Quotient (IQ)} = \text{MA/CA} \times 100$$

1912—Gestalt Psychology
1913—Carl Jung Analytical psychology
1924—JB Watson, an early behaviorist, publishes behaviorism
1935—Thematic Apperception Test
1942—Counseling and psychotherapy
1942—Minnesota multiphasic personality inventory
1951—Carl Rogers—humanistic perspective
1953—BF Skinner, Behavior perspective
1954—Abraham Maslow published motivation and personality, developing the concept of self-actualization

1957—Leon Festinger published a theory of cognitive dissonance, producing major impact on social psychology
1968—First Doctorate in Psychology (Psy.D) awarded (from the University of Illinois)
1973—APA endorsed the Psy.D degree for professional practice in PSYCHOLOGY
1985—Increasing emphasis on cognitive perspective
1990—Greater emphasis on multiculturalism and diversity
2000—New subfields develop such as clinical neuropsychology and evolutionary psychology.

DEFINITIONS

In order to define the subject psychology, it is necessary to know the **philosophical meaning**. The ancient philosophers defined psychology as "study of the mind".

Psychology is the scientific study of people, the mind, and behavior. It is both thriving academic discipline and vital professional practice (The British Psychological Society).

Psychology: The scientific study of the behavior of individual and their mental processes (American Psychological Association).

Both these definitions tell us that psychology is fundamentally concerned with understanding behavior.

Sir W Hamilton: Psychology is defined as a science about the phenomena of the mind, conscious subject, or self.

William Mc. Doughall—1949: Psychology is a science, which aims to give us better understanding and control of the behavior of the organism as a whole.

NL Munn—1967: Psychology is a science and properly trained psychologist is a scientist or at least a practitioner who uses scientific methods or information resulting from scientific investigation.

Crow and Crow: Psychology is the study of human behavior and human relationships.

Psychiatry deals with the medical specialization on mental illness and psychologist deals with common principles without using drugs toward their recovery from simple mental illness.

SCOPE OF PSYCHOLOGY

The subject psychology is regarded to be as science of behavior of animals and human beings.

The subject psychology has wide scope and is applicable to different organizational sectors such as employment, industries, education, and personality development. These are the popular areas where psychology is applied in the treatment of mental and emotional problems.

The field of psychology studies, describes, and explains the behavior of living organisms. Psychologists are interested to know the differences of behavior of people and influence of heredity and environment. The subject psychology has wide scope **(Fig 1.2)** and is applicable theories of psychology study of behavior.

BRANCHES OF PURE PSYCHOLOGY

General Psychology

General psychology is relatively a large area of psychology which deals with the fundamental rules, principles, and theories of psychology to study of behavior of normal human beings.

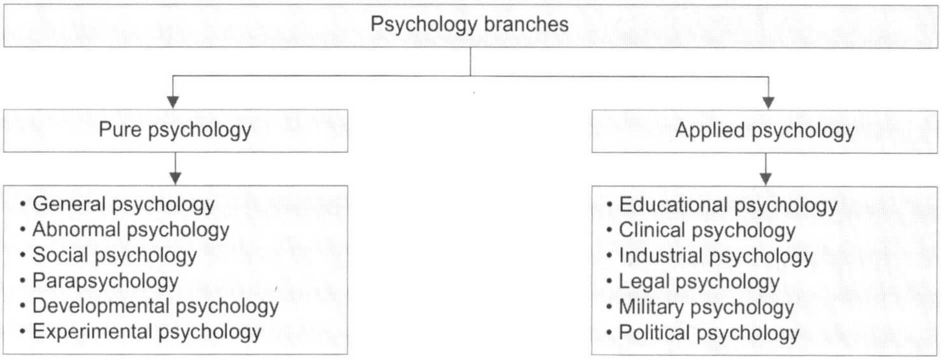

Fig. 1.2: Psychology branches

It also studies the developmental attitudes on their motivational and emotional behavior. It concentrates on attention, perception, thinking, memory, learning abilities, attitudes, and motivational and emotional behavioral process of human behavior.

Abnormal Psychology

Abnormal psychology is the branch of psychology that studies abnormal behavior, emotional thoughts, aggressive attitudes, suicidal tendencies, and some other mental disorders of behavior. The mental disorders are treated by profession with specialization in psychiatry and clinical psychology in mental hospitals. The abnormal cases need hospitalization for the recovery of severe mental disorders.

Social Psychology

This branch of social psychology deals with the group behavior and interactions of people in the society. Its study depends on social circumstances, people's desires, interest, social distances, and prejudices among the public of society.

The subject studies the social dynamics and their influences in the developmental process of society. It also focuses to know the differences in social relations, their maladjustment in working areas and families, etc.

The subject social psychology observes the changes in group behavior by researching on crime and causes of motivating perspectives and attitudes of criminal behavior, and helps the government in managing laws and amendments.

The knowledge and study of social psychologists is useful in survey of students and parents toward the development of society and reformation of social changes in public. The branch of social psychology has greater importance in projecting facts and their consequences in social groups of the society.

Parapsychology

Psychology is the scientific study of interactions between living organisms and their external environment.

It is identified as pseudoscience by the overwhelming majority of mainstream scientists.

Developmental Psychology

Developmental psychology can be defined as discipline in describing the changes occurring in human growth from infant to old age according to the necessities of individuals. It is further subdivided into branches like child psychology, adolescent, adult, and old age psychology. Developmental psychologists try to understand complex behaviour by studying their beginner and the orderly ways in which they change or develop over the life span **(Fig 1.3)**.

Developmental psychologists depend on behavioral process and study the factors of human growth. It is divided into subfields of child psychology, adolescent psychology, and adult psychology. The behavioral changes occurring in different stages from infant to maturity are stated in Figure 1.3 in developmental process of human growth.

Experimental Psychology

This branch of psychology studies the ways and means of carrying out psychological experiments by using scientific methods and describes the methods in an experimental way with proof. The experiments are conducted on animals, birds, and human beings by controlling them in laboratories to study their mental process of behavior. It helps for better understanding of human mind and behavior.

Experimental psychologist focuses his research on behavior of human beings and studies the process of learning, memory, sensation, perception, and motivation.

Comparative Psychology

This field studies the behavior of animals and compares and contrasts it with human beings. This branch also compares the differences of other individuals in social structure.

Pavlov's (1897/1902) studies of classical conditioning in dogs and Skinner's studies of operant conditioning in rats are therefore seen as providing insights into human psychology.

Another application of comparative psychology is in the study of child development.

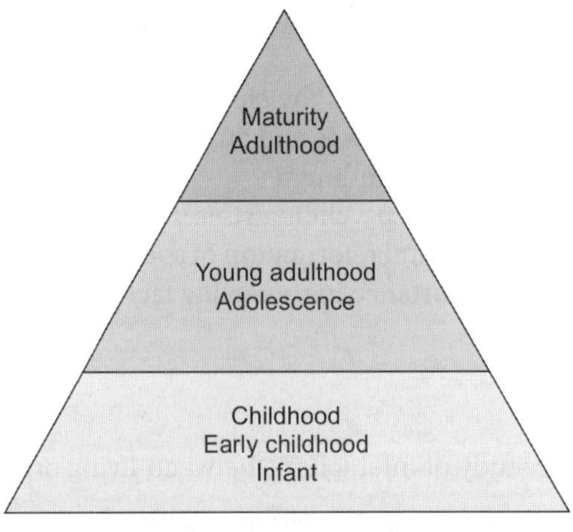

Fig. 1.3: Developmental stages

Cognitive Psychology

Cognition is a mental process in getting awareness of thinking process by experiences and sensations. It deals with the behavioral process of attention, perception, learning, thinking, intelligence, memory, and attitudes of different groups. It has been an integrated study of educational, social, personal, emotional abnormal development process in psychological process. It helps in problem solving and communicational process of human beings.

BRANCHES OF APPLIED PSYCHOLOGY

Applied psychology is a branch in psychology which utilizes the concepts of psychology in solving the practical problems prevalent in various fields.

Educational Psychology

Educational psychology is a branch of applied psychology, which tries to apply the psychological principles, theories, and techniques to human behavior in educational situations. This knowledge is useful in improving learning processes in teaching. The experts from this branch are more essential in dealing with physically handicapped children. The slow learners are also benefited by applying techniques to improve their education. The personality traits and the effectiveness of the teacher, the student-teacher relationship, the attitudes, etc., are the important perspectives in education psychology.

Clinical Psychology

Clinical psychology describes the causes of mental illness and abnormal behavior of a patient and suggests treatment toward social adjustment of family and environment. In other words, clinical psychology is the scientific study and application of psychology in order to understand, prevent, and manage to lead life. It helps to motivate the distress person in modification of human behavior.

Clinical psychologists are employed in hospitals, clinics, and private practice. They often work closely with other specialists in the field of mental health.

The psychologists mostly work with psychiatrists in this field.

Counseling Psychology

Counseling psychology is a psychological specialty. It helps in career development and prevention of ill-health. It strengthens the abilities or skills of client for healthy development of human life. In modern days, people are facing difficulty in changing environment and social conditions in both personal and social life. The counseling psychologist helps in adjustment of marital problems for the well-being of the family by profession. Their knowledge helps clients to overcome from stressful situation which causes depressions and frustrations in day-to-day life. The counseling psychologists are appointed in education institutions to provide counseling to students in career development.

In 1983, Government of India launched a scheme of family counseling centers (FCC). It is being implemented by Central Social Welfare Board through voluntary organizations all across the country. The main goal of this field is to provide preventive and rehabilitation services to women and families who were victims of harassment and family maladjustments through crisis intervention and systematic counseling.

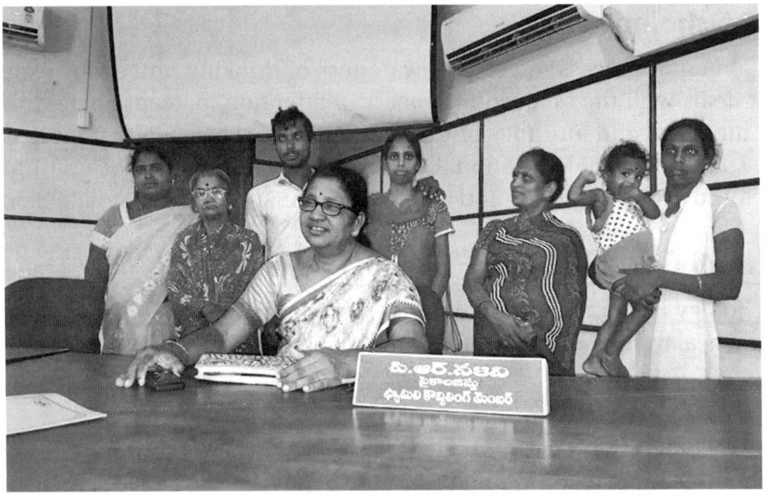

Fig. 1.4: Compromised family after family counseling by support of women police station

The police department started a special women's grievance **(Fig. 1.4)** redressed cell to address family issues that women face in their marital life. The family counseling members will help the marital couples while facing strained relations, marital discord, and protect the family to discuss their problems and find solutions to their marital and family problems.

The counseling establishes mutual solution to disputes. The counseling psychologists conduct counseling in two or four sessions for the couple and relatives based on the cases; 75% of couples compromise after counseling sessions by some of the women police stations.

Industrial Psychology

The branch of applied psychology tries to seek application of the psychological principles, theories, and techniques for the study of human behavior and relation to industrial environment. The workload, insufficient income, lack of rest, and lack of recreations may lead to distress in employees of organization.

The study of organization psychology helps in implementation of policies in administration and coordination between employees and managing group. Its knowledge helps to develop organizations in improving business, etc. This field suggests management in creating recreation and benefits to the working group for healthy development in both sides.

The appointment of industrial psychologists in industries reduces the problems and quarrels among the workers for long duration in working in the same organization.

Legal Psychology

Legal psychology tries to study the behavior of various areas of clients like criminals and their psychological conditions with principles and techniques. The knowledge of legal psychology makes them to know the causes of criminal behavior attitudes by analyzing psychological, emotional, and social causes of their behavior.

Legal psychologists study the basic social, cognitive principles and apply techniques in finding the causes of delinquent behavior. The expertness of this branch makes them easy to take legal decisions by providing safety and peace in the society.

The term "legal psychology" recently came into usage on legal issues. It is primarily focusing on the way to differentiate experimental methods from clinically-oriented forensic psychology. Psychology and law became a field of study in the year 1960. It is providing education to psychologists on legal issues in a psychological view.

Military Psychology

The American Psychology Association has recognized that military psychology has very important role in military administration. The domain of military psychology is the conduct of research or practice of psychological principles within a military environment.

The subject of military psychology is very useful in assessing the behavior of soldiers of courage, functional atmosphere toward the welfare of nation, and creation of self-confidence in working environment.

Political psychology is an interdisciplinary academic field dedicated to understanding principles and techniques in studying politics and changing trends. The psychological awareness is necessary in motivating people to particular party in gaining support from the public. The political survey helps in achieving success or failure in winning votes from the public. It also helps in tolerating the failures in their political atmosphere.

Political Psychology

This branch of psychology focuses on psychological principles and techniques in study of political matter and administration. Political psychology aims to understand interdependent relationships between individuals and contexts that are influenced by beliefs, motivation, perception, cognition, information processing, learning strategies, socialization, and attitude formation.

The political psychologists study the foundations, dynamics, and outcomes of political behavior using cognitive and social explanations.

School Psychology

According to American Psychological Association, school psychology is a general practice and health service provider specialty of professional psychology that is concerned with the science and practice of psychology with children, youth, families; learners of all ages; and the schooling process.

The branch of school psychology is based on development skills of children in learning, intelligence, memory, etc. It helps to improve their knowledge toward social environment, education, etc. Implementation of technical skills is also used to measure attitude and interest by study of school psychology.

SUB-FIELDS IN PSYCHOLOGY

The American Psychological Association is focused on brain and its influence of human behavior. It is also focused on physical responses of habits in measuring of aspects in human personality development.

The American Psychological Association is focusing on everything from how the brain physically responds to habits and interactions and how to measure aspects of personality and behavior.

The knowledge of psychology is used to improve functioning in schools and workplace communities and manage safer plans in leading peaceful life.

1. Aviation

Aviation psychologists study all aspects related to pilot performance in order to increase safety.

2. Biological and Physiological

This area of study focuses on the physical processes of and correlations with psychology.

3. Consumer

This field studies how consumers interact with products and services, often to help companies better sell those products and services.

4. Child Psychology

The branch of child psychology studies the behavior of children and their cognitive feelings of social circumstances.

5. Family

This field examines and seeks to improve family and marital relationships.

6. Forensic

This psychology is when psychologists use their expertise for legal or criminal cases.

7. Psychometric and Quantitative

Psychometrics psychology deals with tests and experiments that measure personality and intelligence.

8. Sports

This is the study of psychology that can be used to improve performance and motivation in athletes.

PSYCHOLOGY RELEVANCE TO NURSING

The subject psychology is relevant to nursing in understanding human behavior to achieve success in their professional life.

Psychology is the science which deals with the way in which our minds work. It also deals with emotional feelings, thoughts, intelligence, and interactions. Psychology has become an integral part in various health professions. The study of human behavior has great value to a student nurse in a number of ways.

The Importance of Study of Psychology in Nursing (Fig. 1.5)

1. Psychology Helps in Understanding Herself

Psychology will help nurses to understand human behavior of patients in diagnosis and treatment of illness. It helps by providing self-confidence in managing healthy social relations. It will be helpful in solving conflicts in different social circumstances.

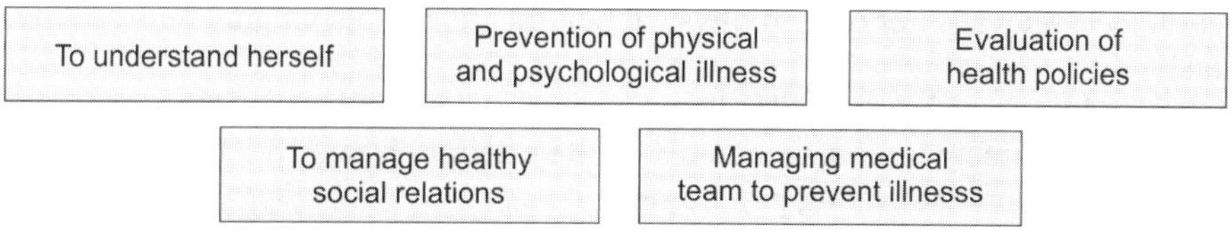

Fig. 1.5: The importance of study of psychology in nursing

Psychology will help nurses to understand the problematic situations properly and also helps to understand the people related to nursing care either directly or indirectly, and seek their cooperation in managing her responsibilities in their professional life.

Nurses' performance is task oriented while dealing with mental retarded group. In educational sector, the nurses' performance of schools in understanding children's behavior and making them to cooperate for treatment. Sometimes they have to work with physically disabled group.

2. Prevent Physical and Psychological Illness

The study of psychology subject by a nurse helps in assessment of physical and psychological problems. She can help to make them normal by using simple health tips to control and prevent psychological problems in primary level. It is helpful to become normal from physical illness.

3. Evaluation of Health Policies

The nurse can evaluate the psychological condition of the patient by study of psychology. The nurse can educate the patient in motivating skills in modification of behavior. The nurse can understand the weakness of patient in management of friendly relations to assess the crisis of illness. The nurse promotes the family members of the patient in awareness of insurance schemes for treatment. The nurse helps in changing attitudes of the patient who are weak in decision-making and feel difficult to reach their expectations.

4. To Manage Healthy Social Relations

The study of psychology helps nurses to understand the problems of patient's family relations, marital problems, children in families, and in-laws and protect old-age group in diagnosis and treatment. The psychological knowledge in emotional problems to manage healthy relations by applying relaxation techniques to manage healthy social relations among the members in society.

5. Managing Medical Team in Prevention of Illness

In team work, the nurse has more influence in recovery of illness. It is also major responsibility in health team profession. The nurse may face problems in tackling the patient toward success in treatment of the patient. The lack of proper medical facilities, noncooperation of health team members may cause for longevity of treatment. The good medical facilities can prevent illness.

So the knowledge of psychology will help the nurse to understand the problems and needs of patients in promotion of good health. She can understand the motives, attitudes, perceptions, and personality characteristics of patients in a better way. This makes the patient to attain quick relief and cure from sickness.

Psychology is relevant not only in physical healthcare, but also highly relevant in the field of mental health.

The knowledge of psychology will help nurses to understand abnormal behavior of mentally retarded patients. Nurses working in mental hospitals definitely need full knowledge of general, abnormal, clinical, and counseling psychology.

The psychological knowledge helps nurses in understanding the health problems of communities and causes for sickness.

It helps in easy understanding of social conditions: The subject knowledge of psychology helps nurses in assessment of weakness and illness by observations of social environment of family, marital relations, and children. The nurses in community health centers may help people by recognizing the mental illness in the early stages and convince them to take appropriate treatment. They can also help people to prevent mental illness by appropriate guidance to deal with stress, anxiety, and other life problems.

One of the role models to nursing profession: Florence Nightingale (1820–1910) **(Fig. 1.6)** was given the nickname "The Lady with the Lamp" and she worked hard to improve the education of nurses. She rendered her services to the soldiers in the war field. She is most well-known for her work during the Crimean war.

The study and knowledge of subject psychology helps the nurse in reducing the tension and worry on serious causes for illness of the patient. Good nursing care also depends upon the ability of a nurse to understand the situations properly, and also in obtaining cooperation of other people concerned. Psychology will help nurses to understand the critical situations related to nursing care either directly or indirectly. The coordination of medical team and their efficiency will help in speedy recovery of the patients.

The knowledge of psychology motivates the nurse, thus helping in alerting communities in prevention of diseases. It also helps in promotion of psychological awareness and prevention of mental illness, suicide, etc.

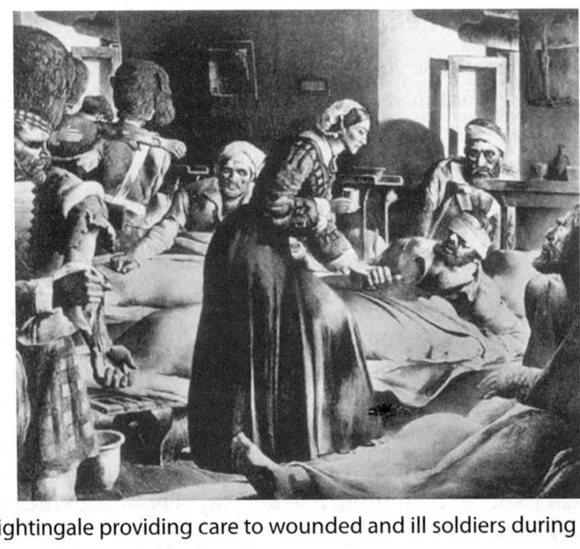

Fig. 1.6: Nightingale providing care to wounded and ill soldiers during Crimean war

CAREER IN PSYCHOLOGY

Psychologists are working as counselors **(Fig. 1.7)** in academic settings, clinical psychologists with specialization of clinical psychology in hospitals, family counseling members in women police stations, juvenile homes, counseling psychologist in industries, and other business settings.

The motivational programs of psychology help public who are facing frustration, depression, etc. It is also bringing awareness of guidance and counseling.

Psychologist has greater role in educational sector to manage healthy and friendly relations among classmates in institutes.

Natural calamities: The psychological awareness supports the disturbed people by natural calamities in promotion of self-confidence and promotion of health.

War: Treat issues such as post-traumatic stress syndrome, and provide counseling to the families of soldiers.

Industries: In industries, the psychologist functions on bringing rapport between employees and management on stress-related issues, planning of work, physical fitness, work load, relaxation techniques, insurance facilities, etc.

Business: In business field the common issues profit and loss of the organization effects on both professional and personal life. The loss of the business may be the cause for substance abuse, suicide, etc. The awareness of psychologists may guide the client to tolerate frustrating moments to cross the miserable situations.

Psychologists are working in mental health centers, hospitals, educational institutions, prisons, industries, etc.

Some of the nongovernment organizations are encouraging the government to appoint one psychologist and nurse in every girl's residential to provide psychological support in adolescent age. Recently, Government took decision in appointment of one male and one female psychologist in every Navodaya educational institute of India. These psychologists support the psychologically weak child in promoting mental health.

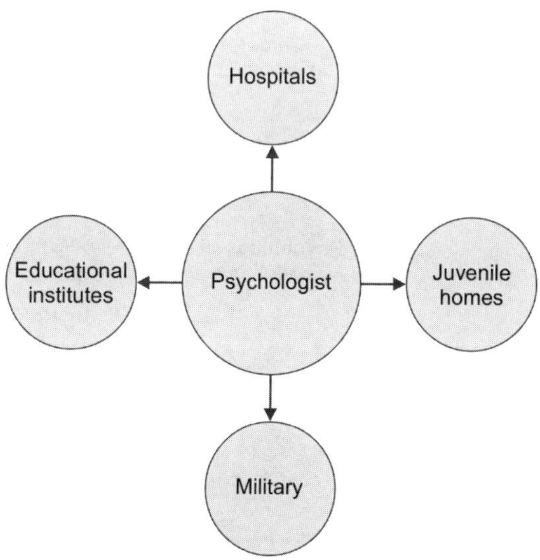

Fig. 1.7: Working places of psychologists

The study of psychology helps in understanding human thoughts and right decision making for well-being of individuals and groups. Psychology helps in examining human behavior in setting of crime, sports, business and clinical health.

Psychological knowledge allows the human being helps in promotion of health. This knowledge helps in decision-making in different working areas. The science of psychology helps to tackle emotional disturbances in individuals and makes them to become normal adults.

Psychological studies have also aided in drug development and the ability to diagnose various diseases (such as Alzheimer's and Parkinson).

Psychology is the study of people's behavior, performance, and mental operations. It also refers to the application of the knowledge, which can be used to understand events, treat mental health issues, and improve education, employment, and relationships.

This psychological knowledge can help in decision-making and choosing right choice. It also helps in time management, setting goals to achieve success in day-to-day incidents.

The psychological knowledge can be observed in different situations of our daily life. The psychological awareness helps in good family relations, social environment, and organizing skills to lead life **(Fig. 1.8)**.

METHODS OF PSYCHOLOGICAL ASSESSMENT

1. Introspection method
2. Observational method
3. Experimental method
4. Clinical method or case study method
5. Survey method
6. Interview method.

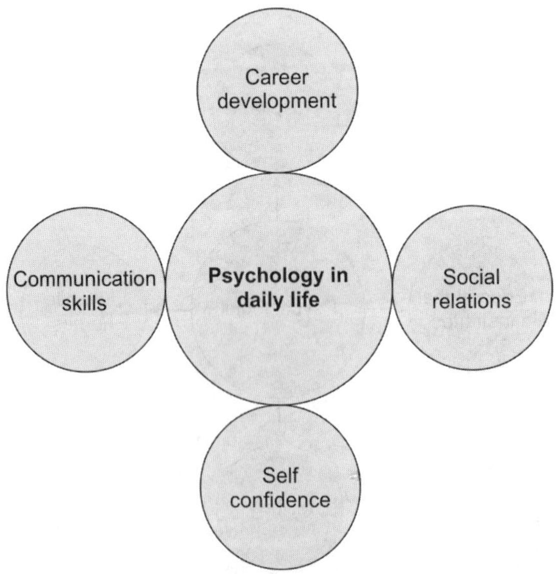

Fig. 1.8: Process of psychology in everyday life

1. Introspection Method

Introspection is also called as self-observational process. In this method, there is no necessity of laboratory or experiments to know the results of the treatment. It is difficult to use this method among children and mentally retarded group. It is an old method mostly used by philosophers in assessing philosophical views.

Introspection method gives direct, immediate results with facts of mental processes. It helps in changing methods of treatment by observing the immediate results of recovery.

2. Observational Method

The method of introspection was replaced by careful observation of human and animal behavior.

Observational method is commonly used by psychologists, behavioral scientists, and social scientists to observe the subjects in natural atmosphere.

The direct and indirect observations both are applicable in conducting the experiment by performing tasks on living organisms. The accurate results are possible by observational method in laboratories.

The observational method helps in understanding emotional changes in human behavior. Nurses can report the patient's temperature, pulse, restlessness, and gestures by using this method. It is more useful to study on children behavior.

3. Experimental Method

In this method, psychologist conducts experiments on living organism to notice learning, memory, forgetting, and many other mental activities. The result of this method is more reliable and variable.

Sometimes they may feel difficult to get cooperation from animals, etc. All experiments are conducted under controlling process. The controlling system is not good. It is very difficult to assess the results. In this method, the plans are proved by experimental process than observational method. It is also expensive to implement the process. Sometimes it takes long duration to confirm results by conducting experiments.

4. Clinical Method or Case Study Method

The main aim of this method is to treat the mentally retarded group by specialized professionals such as clinical psychologists or psychiatrists. It is very difficult and expensive to maintain clinical settings. A variety of techniques are employed including personal interviews, psychometric tests, direct observation, and maintenance of records of case study. They need trained medical team to manage the mentally ill patients. The specialists in this method try to understand patient's fears, anxieties, worries, tensions, and frustrations to achieve success in treatment. Sometimes they need more hospitalization for recovery of severe mental disorders. They need case histories and social interactions toward treatment of mental illness. Psychiatry specialization in nursing education is eligible to work in mental hospitals and other mentally retarded patients.

5. Survey Method

A survey is designed to collect information from different categories of people in a society. The public opinion has more value before confirming the policies on human behavior of different ages. The survey conducted to know the opinion on particular aspect. They may use rating system, comparison, spiritual thoughts, and beliefs and superstitions in survey method. In modern society, they are using mobiles by SMS (short message services) to know the public opinion.

6. Interview Method

This method is used by researchers by face to face contacts by observing the individual's feeling, gestures, and body movement by conducting interview. It is easy to notice psychological and emotional behavior of the human beings. This method useful to recruit employees to assess their interest, attitude and skill for the development of Government organizations.

According to PV Young, "Interview is not a simple way to conversation between an investigator and informant. Gestures, glances, facial expressions, and pauses often reveal subtle feelings."

The main objective of interview method is to collect information about unknown fact of the subject and inner feelings.

CONCLUSION

The study of psychology and its historical background helps nurses in understanding evolution of psychology as a science and subject and understand the significance of change in beliefs and superstitions in a developing healthy society.

The study of the knowledge of psychology guides in diagnosis and treatment of patients. The scope of psychology is wide and understanding the meaning of each branch helps the nurse to grow professionally.

The various methods used in assessing the psychological aspects are helpful in understanding psychological behavior of individual and group of people. The study of methods in psychology helps in diagnosis and treatment of the patient. The study of psychology is essential to various health professionals of India and around the world.

QUESTIONS

Essay Questions

1. Define psychology and discuss its scope with special reference to nursing.
2. Explain the methods used in the study of psychology.
3. Define psychology. Explain the applications of psychology to the other fields.
4. Define psychology and what are the different methods used in the study of psychology. Critically evaluate them.

Short Notes

1. Experimental method.
2. Explain any two branches of psychology.
3. Case study method.
4. Why should a student nurse study psychology?

Brief Questions

1. Child psychology.
2. List the branches of psychology.
3. Write the meaning of introspection method.
4. Define parapsychology.
5. Relevance of psychology in nursing.
6. List down the scope of psychology in nursing.
7. Definition of psychology and its methods.

Fill in the Blanks

1. ________________is defined as "The scientific study of behavior and mental processes." (Psychology)
2. The term psychology is derived from -------------words. (Greek)
3. The branch which deals with general principles of psychology is ------------- (general psychology).
4. First psychology laboratory was established by -----------(Wilhelm Wundt).
5. ________________ founded the School of Psychoanalysis. (Sigmund Freud)
6. The branch of ________________ deals with the behavior of the children from birth to the beginning of the period of adolescence. (Child psychology)
7. ________________ deals with extrasensory perception, cases of re-birth, telepathy, and allied problems. (Parapsychology)
8. The term ________________ refers to all processes by which the sensory input is transformed, reduced, elaborated, stored, recovered, and used. (cognition)
9. ________________ deals with mental, emotional, and abnormal behavior of the people. (Clinical psychology)
10. ________________ studies the way people change or develop physically, emotionally, intellectually, and socially throughout their lives. (Developmental psychology)
11. Psychiatry deals by the medical specialization on ________________ and ________________ deal with common principles without using drugs toward their recovery from mental illness. (mental illness, psychologists)

Multiple Choice Questions

1. Psychology is ....
   a. Study of behavior
   b. Study of human health
   c. Study of disease
2. The term psychology was derived from .... words.
   a. Latin
   b. France
   c. Greek
3. The branch which deals with general principles of psychology is ....
   a. Comparative psychology
   b. Developmental psychology
   c. General psychology

4. Greek philosophers defined psychology as psychology as ....
   a. Study of soul
   b. Study of mind
   c. Both (a) and (b)
5. First psychology lab was established by........................
   a. Sigmund Freud
   b. Wilhelm Wundt
   c. Max Wertheimer

Answers

1. a	2. c	3. c	4. c	5. c

CHAPTER 2

Biology of Behavior

Learning Objectives

- Body mind relationship: Modulation process in health and illness
- Genetics and behavior: Heredity and environment
- Brain and behavior: Nervous system, neuron and synapse
- Association cortex, right and left hemispheres
- Psychology of sensations
- Muscular and glandular controls of behavior
- Nature of behavior of the organism/ integration of responses

The biology of behavior means functioning process of body and mind. In the process of cognition, function of body, sensations have key role on human behavior. The changes of physical and psychological conditions occur by influence of body mind coordinations in human beings.

The behavioral changes depend on condition of both physical and psychological in coordination of body mind relation of individuals. It influences in ability of thinking process and loss of sensations in human behavior.

Some of the physical disorders lead to cancer and imbalance of heartbeats.

Behavioral psychologists believed that psychology is concerned with observation on stimulus and responses.

BODY-MIND RELATIONSHIP: MODULATION PROCESS IN HEALTH AND ILLNESS

Mind fills with various mental processes like observation, thinking, reasoning, memory, intelligence and judgment. Mind is based as the function of body and it is not existing apart from the body. The human developmental process depends on the activities of body and mind. Mental functions and physical states affect each other. The health related problems and disease that come from psychological based on physical conditions of human being.

Sometimes the severe mental disorders lead to higher death rates of individuals. It also affects general health by heart diseases and cancers.

The mind programs the physical activities in body like in computer. The new ideas created in brain for progress of psychological strength to face conflicts and frustration, etc. The psychological strength supports human in managing stress and emotional changes in preventions of mental illness. Both body and mind are coordinated for health condition of individual.

Body is represented by physical states and bodily functions. Lack of rest, work load, irregular diet effects on functioning of body, and also leads to mental stress.

Rise in blood pressure leads to mental excitement. Sudden emotions causes mental imbalance. Hyperthyroidism leads to excitement and hypothyroidism causes lethargy. The emotional imbalance effects on cardiac attacks, ulcers, cancer, etc. Constipation leads to irritation, depression, restlessness, and overexcitement. Thyroid gland has very important function in the development of physical structure as well as mental development. The nervous systems and structure of brain has greater role in body and mind functional process. Brain injuries lead to loss of memory and forgetfulness. Forgetting is common in most of the old people. So the improvement in treatment of brain injuries helps to both physical and mental activities of diseased.

The mental disorders caused by noncoordination of mind and body and effects human behavior.

Recently, scientists have speculated that behavioral disorders, such as autism has a biological basis. At the same time, they have been rediscovering the links between stress and health. It shows the powerful mind and body connections through emotional, mental, social, spiritual, and behavioral factors can directly effects on health. Unconscious motivation and conflicts gives rise to many physical complaints and neurotic disorders.

The psychologists help to the depressed people by counseling in primary level of illness. Yoga and meditation is also useful in relaxation from distress.

Some of the useful techniques of psychology helps in modification of behavior in change of harmful habits like smoking, addiction of drugs, etc. It is an altered state of consciousness. Hypnotism can be used to reduce pain, improve attention process of human behavior. Hypnotists are using this technique in clinical practice to reduce smoking, alcohol and gambling.

In ancient days most of the people got peace by meditation. In modern days most of the school children getting healthy by doing yoga, physical exercise to feel free from distress. It is also improving memory and concentration. This process is easy to implement even for senior citizens.

Effect of Drugs on Human Behavior

Drugs which alter consciousness are called psychoactive drugs and act directly upon brain. They can be stimulants, depressants or hallucinogens. Stimulants—Caffeine, nicotine, cocaine, methamphetamine, prescription stimulants etc. Alcohol, barbiturates and marijuana are depressants. Drug addicted patient faces difficulty in modification of behavior. In primary level it can be treated but it effects both physical and mental illness in severity of addiction.

Psychoactive substances often bring about subjective changes in consciousness and mood. Drug Rehabilitation attempts to reduce addiction, through a combination of psychotherapy and psychoactive substances.

The Government implementing restrictions in sales of substances which are harmful to health. Ethical concerns also been raised about over-use of these drugs clinically, and about their marketing by manufacturers.

GENETICS AND BEHAVIOR

Genetics is a branch of biology concerned with the study of genes, genetic variation and heredity in organism. In human behavior most of the characteristics and physical features transmitted by genes. Behavioral genetics deals with understanding both genetics and environment which contributes individual variations in human behavior.

Genes play a major role in transmitting characteristics and structural growth from one generation to another generation. Some other characteristics and influenced by environment. The cognitive processes of learning, intelligence etc. may developed by influence environment. Some of the interests in games and sports may developed by physical energy and social circumstances of individuals.

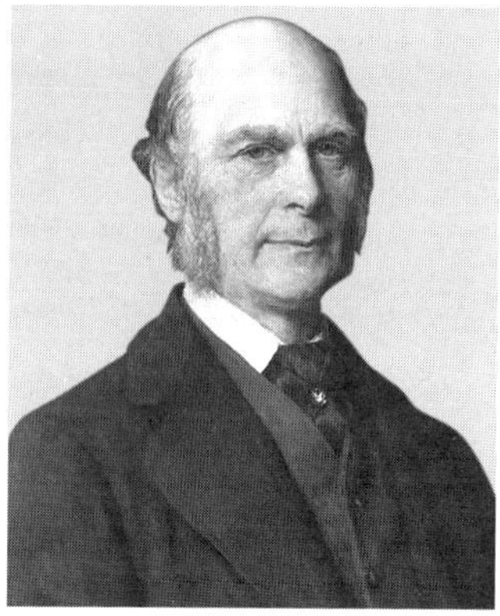

Fig. 2.1: Francis Galton

Transference of the traits was studied scientifically by Gregor Mendel, an Australian monk. He did not know the physical basis for heredity. Mendel observed that organisms inherit transmits via distinct units of inheritance. His work led to the knowledge of dominant and recessive genes in explaining the heredity transmission of traits and related facts about mutation inheritance.

Recently, this field has moved into the area of statistical genetics, with many behavioral geneticists also involved in efforts to identify the specific genes involved in human behavior, and to understand how the effects associated with these genes changes across time, and in conjunction with the environment.

Francis Galton **(Fig. 2.1)** was the first to apply statistical methods to study of human differences and inheritance.

Hereditary is the study of transmission of characters from one generation to another generation and variations in behaviour in individuals of species.

In psychology, this phase lasted for the first half of the 20th century largely because of the overwhelming influence of behaviorism in this field. Later behavioral genetic research focused on quantitative methods.

Mechanism of Heredity

Generally, gene has two alternative forms. The inheritance of trait that is determined by a gene located on one of the sex chromosomes is called sex-linked inheritance.

Deoxyribonucleic acid (DNA) is a chemical compound that contains genetic instructions needed to develop and direct the activities of every organism in the form of a set of chromosomes.

The total DNA from cell is isolated and converted into random fragments of relatively smaller size. Genes that are present X and Y chromosomes are called sex-linked chromosomes. Females have 23 pairs of XX chromosomes. Males have 22 pairs of XX plus two singles represented by X and Y. The probability of inheritance of traits by XY linked genes is similar in both sexes. All female eggs have only one type of chromosomes but sperm cell of the male may contain both X and Y. At the time of conception mother can contribute the same X chromosome, while father contributes either X or Y.

Some DNA is involved in regulating the expression of the genes that code for specific proteins.

A genetic disorder is a disease of syndrome that is cause by abnormality in an individual DNA. A number of disorders in human beings have been found by altered genes or chromosomes.

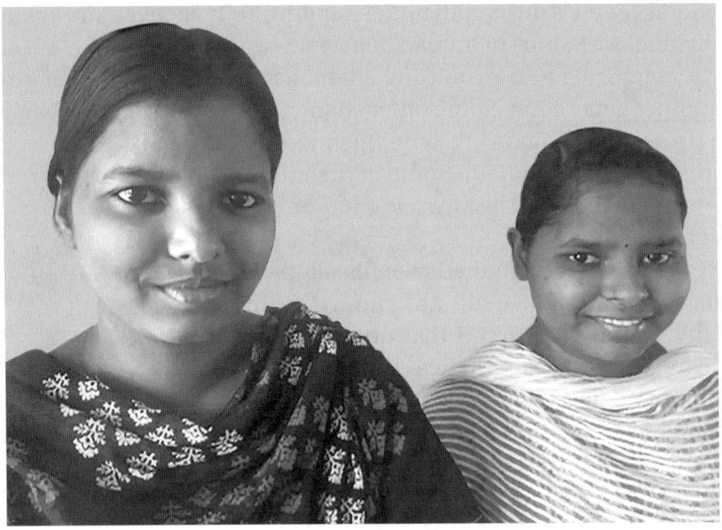

Fig. 2.2: Portrait of Fraternal twins

Color blindness is also sex-linked disorders. X-linked dominant inheritance indicates that a gene is responsible for a genetic disorders located on the X chromosomes.

Fraternal or dizygotic twins **(Fig. 2.2)** born to the same parents are different from each other. However identical or monozygotic twins develop from same sperm and ovum. So they resemble each other.

Many aspects of human behavior and development of physical characteristics like features, height, weight, and skin color influences on genetic basis.

Genetic Interactions

The genetic information is not satisfying in all situations. It is also in controversy in finding facts.

For example, if a child has one tall parent and one short parent, the child may end up splitting the difference by being of average height. In other cases, some genes follow a dominant-recessive pattern. Eye color is one example of dominant-recessive genes at work. The gene for brown eyes is dominant and the gene for blue eyes is recessive. If one parent hands down a dominant brown eye gene while the other parent hands down a recessive blue eye gene, the dominant gene will win out and the child will have brown eyes.

Genetic Environment Interactions

The environment is dominating genetic behavior. For example, exposure to harmful drugs while in utero can have a dramatic impact on later child development. Height is a good example of a genetic trait that can be influenced by environmental factors. The environment may change in habits, intelligence in development of personality. The nutritious diet also influences on human growth of the individual. While a child's genetic code may provide instructions for tallness, the expression of this height might be suppressed if the child has poor nutrition or a chronic illness.

Gene Editing of Human Embryos

Published on August 6th 2017 Indian express, New Delhi: For the first time, genetically modified human embryos have been developed in the US and Kashmir born doctor Sanjeev Kaul has played a lead role in this breakthrough. Scientists have demonstrated an effective way of using gene editing tool to correct a disease causing gene mutation in human embryos and stop it from passing in future generations.

China attempted earlier to alter human embryos using technique called CRISPR Cas9 (Clustered Regularly Interspaced Short Palindromic Repeats) to edit genes to help in removing fatal mutation which leads to heart attacks. CRISPR is a kind of precise molecular scissor the scientists use to edit faulty genes. Only selected embryos were allowed to grow further that too only for few days using the enzyme called Cas9, it is possible to snip a specific target sequence on a mutant gene and in this case it helped remove a fatal mutation that leads to heart attacks.

Genetic Abnormalities

The occurrence of genetic disorder is based on the heredity of certain characteristic features in families. Alternative studies were made to study the family history about the influence of particular trait. A number of disorders found in human beings associated with inheritance. Genetic disorders broadly classified Mendelian and chromosomal disorders. Mendelian disorder causes genetic disease showing Mendelian pattern of inheritance caused by single mutation in the structure of DNA. Disorders are caused by errors in the structure of chromosome cell division.

Researchers suggest that as many as half of all zygotes that form have more than 23 chromosomes, but most of these are spontaneously aborted and never develop into a full-term baby.

Uncertainty, mistrustfulness, insecurity, dependency, responsibility, authoritarianism, jealousy, introversion, and aggressiveness is observed in behavior of first born child.

Most of the second-born children are extroverts, humorous, dependable, and courageous and well-adjusted in their behavior. They will be aggressive, easily distracted, jealousy, inferiority and inadequacy and prone to behavior disorders.

The last-born children are confident, capable, and talented with good nature in their personalities. They are irresponsible, inferior, jealous and happy moments are also common in their characteristics.

Nature-versus Nurture Theory

Nature and nurture are interdependent forces. The branches of psychology are very serious to know the reasons in transmitting of traits from one generation to another depending on either heredity or environment. It is generally believed that human behavior is determined by complex interactions of both nature and nurture. It is difficult to ascertain whether genetics (nature) or the environment (nurture) has strong influence on behavior. Some examples are having strong belief on influence of nature.

Biological psychology tends to stress the importance of genetics and biological influences.

The heredity plays a major role at the time of conception. The most of the heredity factors influences similarities in physical features observable in siblings, and family members by blood relations. Similarities in body structure, voice, color of eyes, complexion, and color of hair depends on hereditary traits. Physical and mental health of mother included in their children by habits, attitudes and interests.

Nurture **(Figs. 2.3A and B)** refers to all the environmental factors influences on physical growth by diet, experiences of social interactions, family, school, and neighborhood, etc. The social agencies have major role nurture theory. The development of personality on human growth from infant to old age depends on different social conditions human environment. The culture is a learned behavior. It is also differing from one society to another. Cultural influences have rapid growth in human behavior.

The heredity and environment influences human behavior, learning behavior, and cultural patterns. The aggressiveness, temperament, intelligence may different in each individual by factors of heredity and environment. The personality traits may be changed by social conditions of stress and frustrations in human life. In this way sometimes environmental conditions leads to severe mental disorders.

The Effect of Heredity on Human Behavior

Heredity refers to the biological process of transmission of certain biological and psychological characteristics from parents to their children through genes.

The close relationship between child physical and moral qualities indicates that both these qualities should have been inherited from the same sources.

Studies by Galton and others history of twins, scientists, judge's, and artist's mental activities are inherited rather than education.

In socialization friends influence is more while growing of age and continuation of friendship are very strong compared to the changes in behavior. So, both are considered toward the development in human growth.

Did You Know?

(From 1905 to 2018). Interest on education in old generation continued for future generation. It helped to get successful professionals like village officer (Karanam) in first two generations, later continued third generation as doctor in medicine, veterinary field, doctorates, professors, bank managers, executives in State and Central Government of India, journalists, authors, advocates, psychologist, and teachers. In fourth generation, IIM degree holders, civil engineers, program officers, veterinary doctors, software professionals, architects, and researchers are working in developed countries and major organizations of U.S.A and U.K in Yahoo, B.B.C, etc. In fifth generation, youths are studying in international universities **(Figs. 2.4A to E)**. It shows both heredity and environment influenced on human behavior.

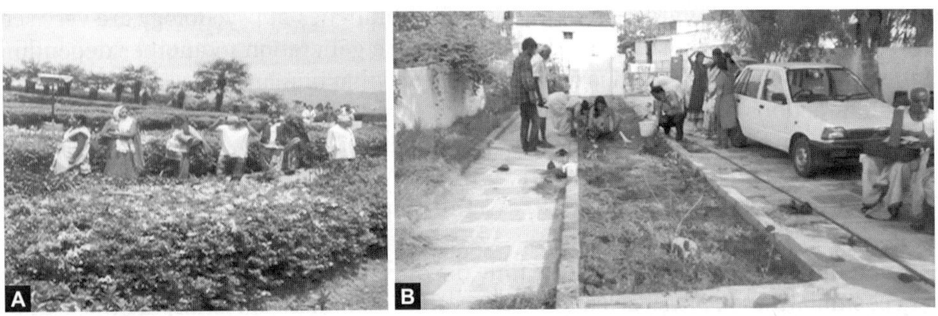

Figs. 2.3A and B: Nature versus nurture

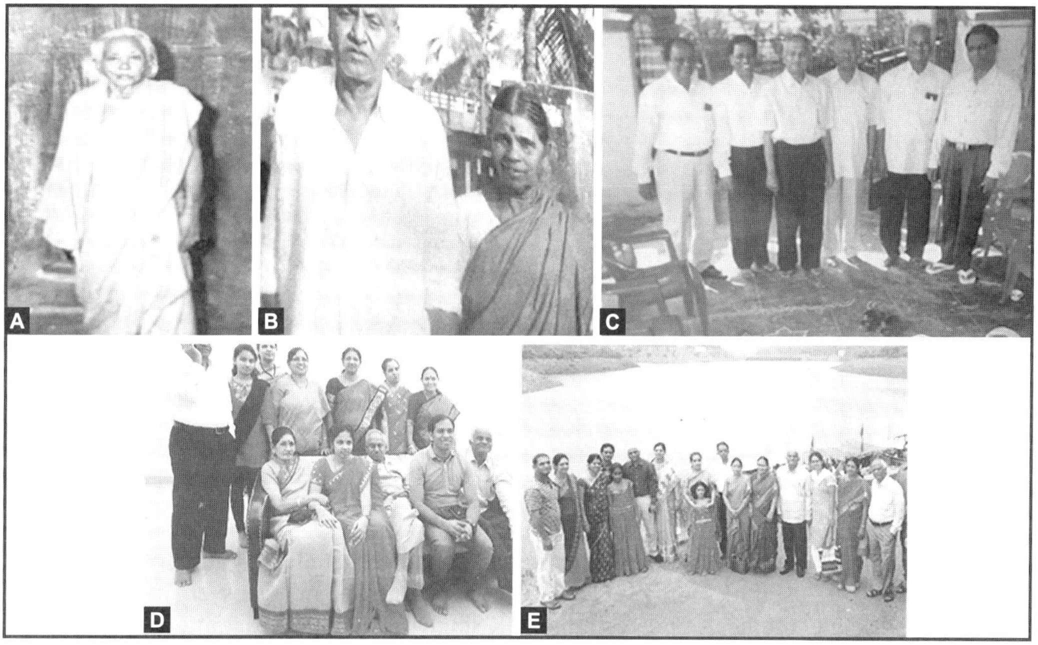

Figs. 2.4A to E: Influence of heredity and environment in fourth generations (1905 to 2018)

In some other families fifty percent are interested in farming, school dropouts in primary level. One is a state rank holder in education with medical profession and some are good in farming and some people are good in dairy development etc.

The above examples studied on personal traits of families on many generations. It is a strong evidence on influence of heredity and environment on human behavior.

Effects of Environment

Environment is surrounded by an organism and exerts directly influence on it. Its role is very important in development of personality.

The neighborhood and social interactions have major role in development of interests, attitudes, temperament, and habits in human behavior.

Hindustan Times, Bahraich, 8th April 1917.

Girl may not have been raised by monkeys (Fig. 2.5): The girl behaved like monkeys, walked on all four walls, ate like animals by picking up food with her mouth, and screened like monkeys to communicate. The girl, possibly eight years, was found in Katarniaghat Wildlife Sanctuary in January, she had matted hair, wounds on her body and wearing underwear when a forest patrol spotted her.

The behavior of this girl prompted people to call the girl Mowgli—after the wolf raised boy protagonist of Rudyard Kipling's iconic children's tale "The Jungle Book".

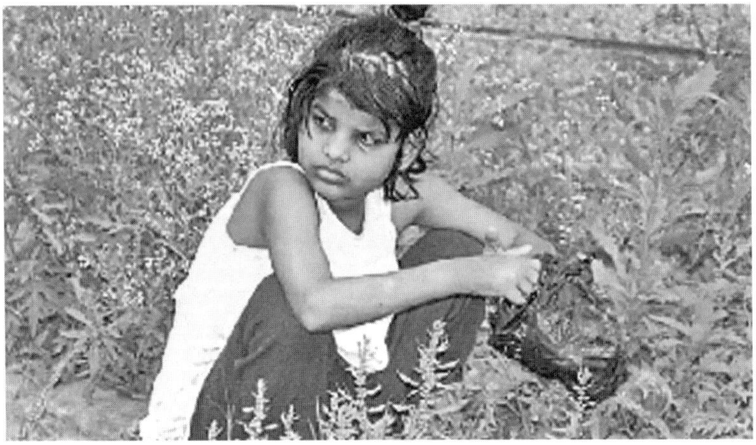

Fig. 2.5: Van Durga was found abandoned in Katarniaghat Wildlife Sanctuary in January

The rescuers brought her to Bahraich district hospital, Uttar Pradesh on January 25th, 2017. Pediatrician KK Verma has doubt that she is a feral child (isolated from human contact from young childhood) raised by monkeys. Doctors believe that she needs psychiatric evaluation and treatment. Chief medical superintendent DK Singh believes the girl imitated the monkeys in the forest.

The girl will be taken to Lucknow for psychiatric evaluation and treatment in accordance with juvenile court order.

The above example appears that influence of environmental is stronger than heredity.

In every generation mix up of blood relations from ancestral traits and environmental factors are common in all individual behavior.

The Brain

The brain is a very important part in body and mind process. In cognitive process, problem solutions, conscious levels, and social behavior depend on functional process of brain. Sometimes the brain injuries affect cognitive process of thinking, memory, etc. The human brain (**Fig. 2.6**) functions on five sense organs and responsible in thinking, feeling, perceiving, and act in the body. The human brain is interconnected by three major components the cerebrum, the cerebellum, and the brain.

The brain is classified mainly into three:

Forebrain is structure of thalamus, hypothalamus and limbic system and cerebrum **(Fig. 2.7)**.

- **Thalamus:** It is superior to the midbrain. It has major role in coordination of center and sensory information. It helps in cognitive process of observing environment by stimulation. It functions as relay station in process of information.
- **Hypothalamus:** It regulates and directs behavior in integrated activities toward adjustment. The brain controls the body by taking help from pituitary gland and nervous system. Centers in hypothalamus have control on main processes of eating, drinking, sleeping, temperature control, and sex.
- **Limbic system:** The limbic system along with hypothalamus is involved in regulation of sexual behavior and expressions of emotional reactions. The limbic system often called the

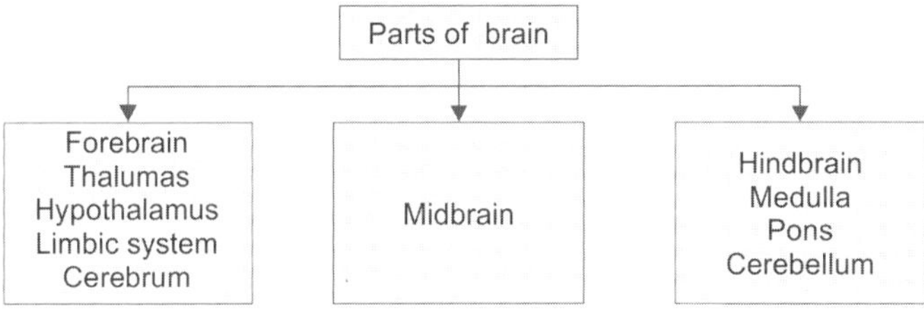

Fig. 2.6: The parts of human brain

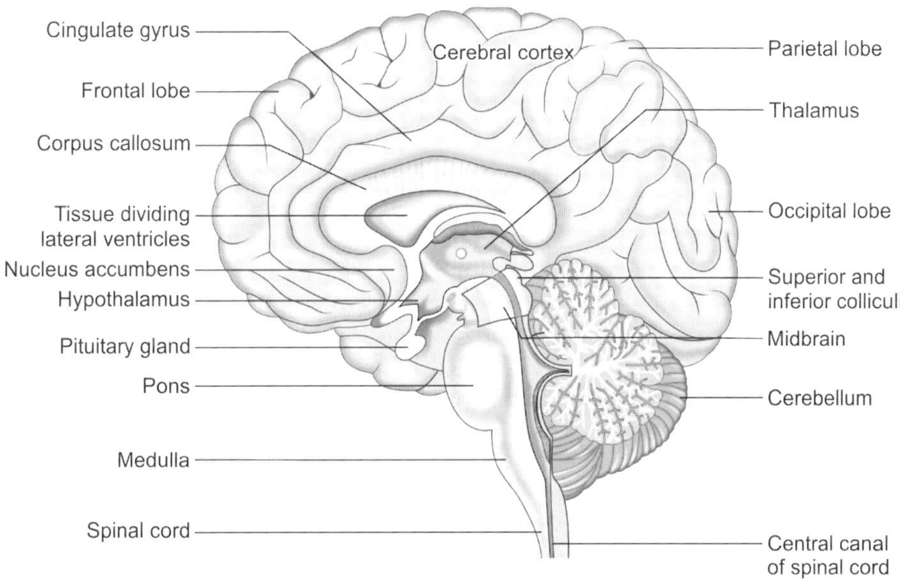

Fig. 2.7: Brain parts

emotional brain, functions in emotional aspects of behavior related to survival memory, smell, pleasure and pain, aggression, affection, etc.

- **The cerebrum:** The cerebrum lies at the top of the brain. It is a largest part of the brain. The cerebrum is covered by sheet of natural tissue known as the cerebral cortex, which envelops other brain organs such as thalamus and hypothalamus.

Right and Left hemispheres, Association Cortex

Cerebrum is divided into two hemispheres—the left and right hemispheres. The cerebrum is covered with thick layer neurons called the cerebral cortex. The area of cerebral cortex and association areas. It controls body movement by coordination and regulation of functions of thinking, reasoning, and problem solving.

Each hemisphere is responsible for the opposite side of the body. The right hemisphere controls movement and receives information from the left side of the body and left hemisphere does the same for the right of the body. The different parts of the cerebrum are connected with different mental functions.

The right hemisphere helps with ability in solving puzzles, picture drawing and noticing objects, etc.

The cerebral cortex is divided into four distinct lobes. The functions of the cerebral cortex (the gray matter) is a mental process of sensory areas as receptors of visual, hearing, taste, touch, pain, and pressure.

Lobe-Functions

The three major lobes **(Fig. 2.8)** located toward the back of the brain are known as the temporal, occipital, and parietal lobes.

1. **Frontal lobe:** The frontal lobe is located at the front of the brain just behind the forehead.
2. **Parietal lobe:** It is located both sides of the head near the top and to the back. It perceives by analyzation and passes information of touch from body. It also integrates and elaborates sensations raised from the body.
3. **Temporal lobe:** Temporal lobe is a large thumb-shaped extension of the cerebral hemispheres located near the temples on either side of the head. A small section at the top of each temporal lobe known as the auditory cortex is responsible for hearing. The temporal lobes are also involved in memory, acquisition, perception and categorization of the objects.
4. **Occipital lobe:** The occipital lobe is in the extreme rear of the cerebral hemisphere at the back of the brain. Injuries in the occipital lobe cause defect in vision, difficulty in identifying of color which leads to abnormalities of perception like illusions and hallucinations.

The midbrain is a sort bridge connecting the forebrain and hindbrain. The midbrain originally a center for coordinating reflexes responses to visual output, has taken an added function related to touch and auditory input. It manages multiple tasks even by distractions.

The hindbrain situated behind and beneath the forebrain. It connects the upper part of the spinal cord with the lowest part of the brain. The hindbrain consists of three parts, i.e. medulla oblongata, cerebellum, and pons.

- **The cerebellum**: It is second largest part of the brain. It consists of two cerebral hemispheres. Each hemisphere consists of three lobes namely anterior, posterior and floccule lobes. The cerebellum is responsible for the control of locomotor movements. Cerebellum is responsible for body balance and the coordination of body movements like dancing, typing, playing, etc.

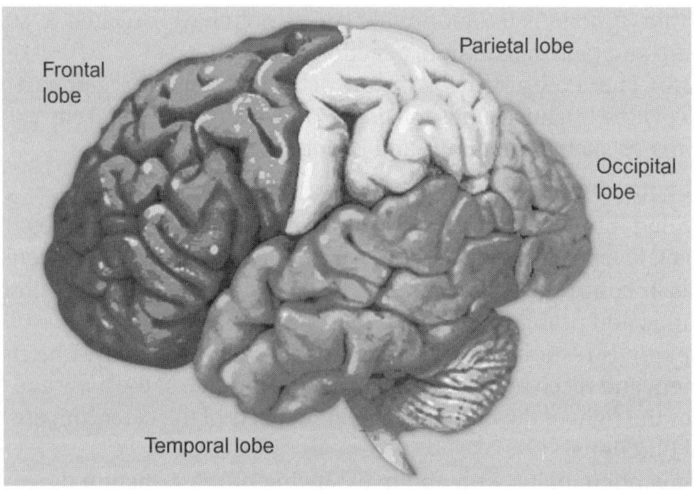

Fig. 2.8: Lobes—location

- **The medulla:** The medulla is an enlargement where the spinal cord enters the brain. It controls the process of transmission of nerve impulses from the lower regions to the other parts of the brain. It controls breathing, digestion, respiration, etc.
- **The pons:** The pons connects the cerebrum at the top of the brain to the topmost section of the hindbrain, the cerebellum. It manages breathing, transmission of impulses from cerebellum to brain areas and coordinates the activities of both sides of the brains. In this way dancing, typing, playing are make easy in performance.

NERVOUS SYSTEM

Nerves system **(Fig. 2.9)** has major role in control, communication, and regulation of body function. The basic unit of nervous system is neuron. It is very important in cognitive processes of thinking, learning, memory, etc. The nervous system classified into types. They are central nervous system and peripheral nervous system.

As per National Institute of health, the central nervous system consists of sensory neurons, ganglia, and nerves that connect to one another and to the central nervous system.

The central nervous system (CNS) consists of brain and spinal cord, which act as the integrating and command centers of nervous system. The spinal cord is cylindrical shaped bundle of nerve fibers that is connected to the brain. They interpret incoming sensory information and issue instructions based on past experience and current conditions.

The spinal nerves are two types—receptors and effectors. The sense organs are called receptors. The muscles and endocrine glands called effectors. The nervous system known as the connecting or integrating mechanism.

The somatic system is both a sensory and motor system. The somatic system consists of nerves that connect the brain and spinal cord with muscles and sensory receptors in the skin. All these sensations normally and consciously perceived. Somatic motor neurons innervate the skeletal muscles and produce voluntary movement.

The sympathetic system controls the processes of digestion, constipation, and the action of glands. It also manages emotional states and reinforce the activities.

The parasympathetic system is connected to the brain and lower portion of the spinal cord. It tends to be active when we are calm and relaxed. The messages conveyed by the nerve fibers of this system direct the organs to do just the opposite of what the sympathetic system had done. It directs body organs to return to a normal state after emergency has passed.

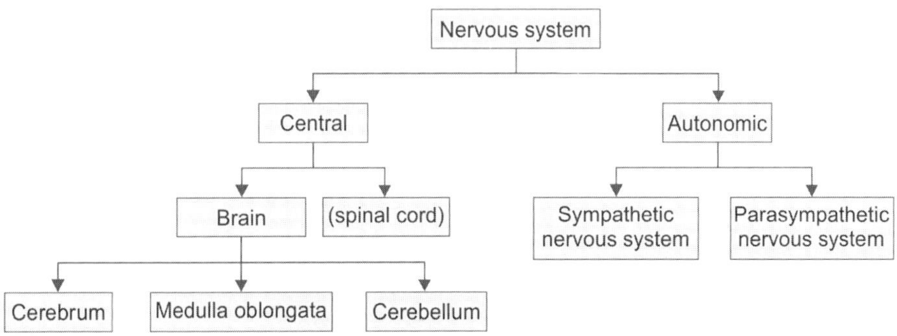

Fig. 2.9: Organization of nervous system

Thus sympathetic and parasympathetic systems are helpful to maintain equilibrium of body functions.

Neurons send signals to other cells through thin fibers called axons, which cause chemicals known as neurotransmitters to be released at junctions called synapse. A synapse gives a command to the cell and the entire communication process typically takes only a fraction of millisecond.

Motor neurons located in the central nervous system **(Fig. 2.10)** or in peripheral ganglia, transmit signals to activate the muscles or glands.

Diagnosing Nervous System Conditions

There are number of tests and procedures to diagnose conditions involving the nervous system. Abnormal tissues such as tumor can be detected because the protons in different types of tissues return to their equilibrium state at different states, tissues such as bones with less water content look different in an MRI (magnetic resonance imaging) **(Fig. 2.11)**. Other standard neurological examinations include CT scan and EEG (electroencephalogram), which records the brain's continuous electrical activity.

The neural substrates of mental image generation were investigated with functional magnetic resonance imaging (MRI). It is medical imaging technique, used in body's natural magnetic properties to produce detailed images any part of the body. It is a sensitive test for the detection of disease. The image produced in MRI in detail and detect changes of structures within the body. A radiologist interprets the images of the body parts and gives diagnostic opinion on patient.

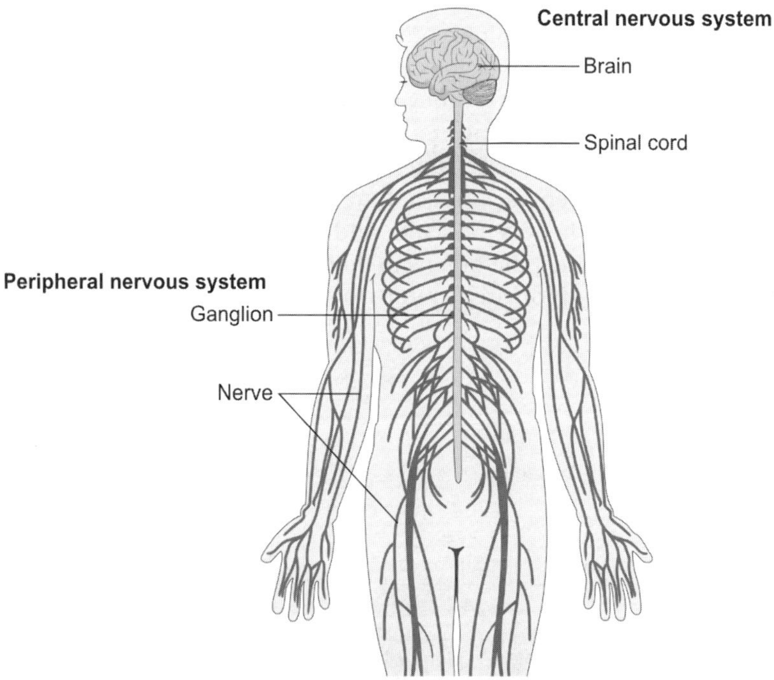

Fig. 2.10: Central nerves system

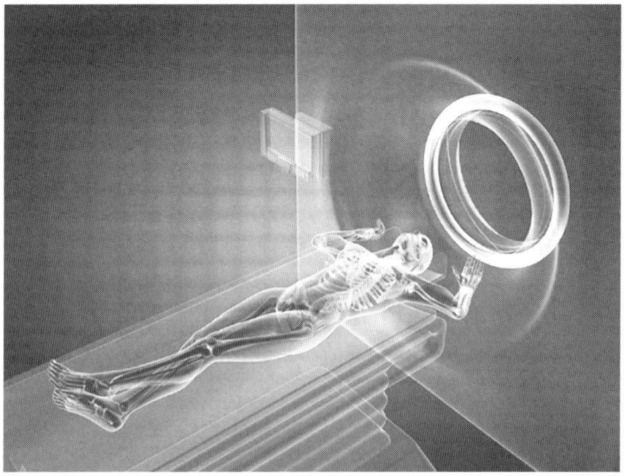

Fig. 2.11: MRI is a medical imaging system used to diagnose health conditions

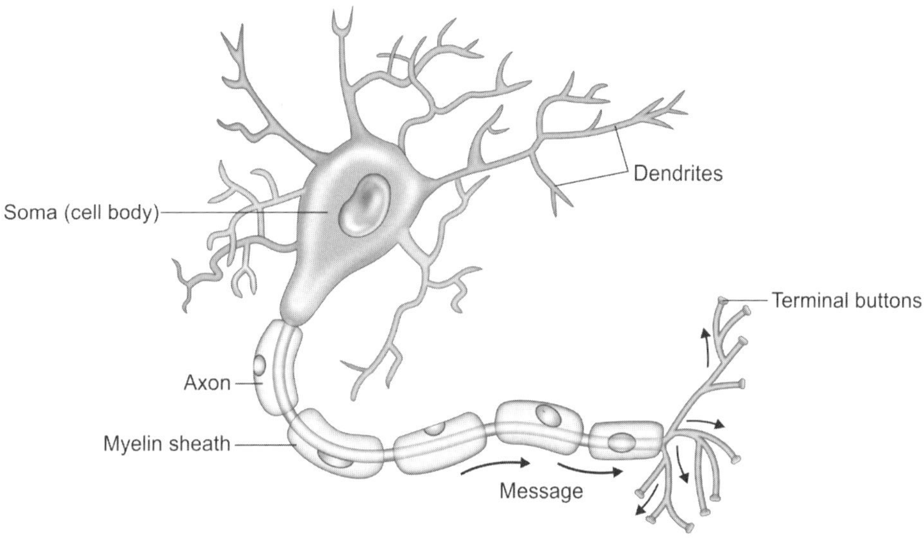

Fig. 2.12: Structure of Neuron

THE NEURON

Neurons **(Fig. 2.12)**, or nerve cells carries information to the nervous system. 90% of all brain neurons are located in the cerebral cortex mainly in the gray matter. Nerve cells have two types of fibers—dendrites, and axon. The dendrites relatively short and have many branches which receive stimulation from other neurons. Axon is long and pass impulses to other neurons or to other muscles and glands. Since the dendrites and the cell body receive information that is conducted along the axon, the direction of transmission is from dendrites to the fine axon tip. Neurons are very important in receiving sensations, controlling muscle movements, regulating digestion, secreting of hormones, and managing mental process of thinking, memory, etc.

Synapse

A nerve impulse is transmitted from one neuron to another through junctions called synapse **(Fig. 2.13).** There are two types of synapses namely electrical and chemical synapses. Neurons are cells that are specialized to pass signals to individuals. In many synapses, the presynaptic part is located on an axon and the postsynaptic part is located on a dendrites or soma. Neurotransmitters are used to carry the signal across the synapse to other neurons. A neurotransmitter is a chemical messenger that caries signals between neurons and other cells of the body.

1. **Epilepsy:** Epilepsy, in which abnormal electrical discharges from brain cells cause seizures.
2. **Parkinson' disease:** It is a progressive disorder of the central nervous system. It affects movement, producing motor symptoms, which include autonomic dysfunction, neuropsychiatric problems and sleep difficulties.
3. **Stroke**: It is rapid loss of brain functions due to disturbance in the blood supply to the brain. This is caused by reduce of blood flow called as hemorrhage. It affects brain inability of movement and speech.
4. **Alzheimer's disease:** It is most common from dementia in elderly. It is progressive neurologic disease of brain causes memory loss, reduces power of intelligence, etc.

Infections such as meningitis, encephalitis and polio, can also affect the nervous system.

The branch of medicine that studies and treats the nervous system is called neurology, and doctors who practice in this field of medicine are called neurologists.

Neurosurgeons perform surgeries involving the nervous system.

PSYCHOLOGY OF SENSATION

The behavior is based on different stimulation exposed by body parts, and feelings of sense organs. The sense organs send messages to brain and influences on mind setting and effects on body. So these sense organs are called as receptors. These sense organs consist of the receptors specialized sensitive cells associated with the endings of sensory nerve fibers and various accessary apparatus and tissues which contribute to the effectiveness with which sense organ functions. Each sense organ has a distinctive and specific function to perform.

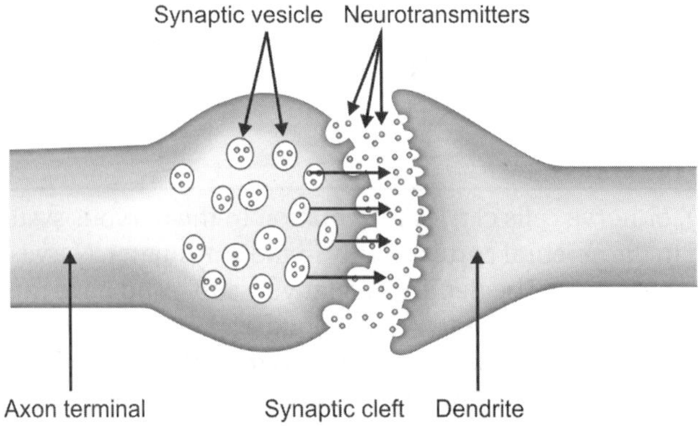

Fig. 2.13: Structure of synapse

The changes in vision, auditory, touch, smell and taste by improper functioning of sense organs. Some of the external environment may cause for physical disorders like pain, sight, deaf, dumb, and allergies.

The function of sense organs proves the importance of brain in experiencing feelings of visual, auditory, touch, taste and smell in daily life. The brain then interprets those neural messages, which allow the brain to experience and make decisions about the environment.

Sensation is the process that allows our brains to take information via our five senses, which can then be experienced and interpreted by the brain.

- **Vision**: The eye is the one of the sense organs in process of vision. In the human visual system, the eye receives physical stimuli in the form of light and sends those stimuli as electrical signals to the brain, which interprets the signals as images.
- **Auditory-hearing:** The ear is the site of reception of two senses namely hearing and equilibrium. The impulses are transmitted by the afferent fibers via the auditory nerves to the auditory cortex of the brain, where the impulses are analyzed in recognizing the sound.
- **Taste:** The sensation of taste passes through taste pores and reaches the taste bud, then the sensation is transferred to the brain resulting in taste experience.
- **Olfaction-Smell:** The olfactory gives humans their senses of smell by collecting odorants from the environment and sending them into neural signals.
- **Motor sensations:** Kinesthetic sensation-sensory inputs which recognize the orientation of the different parts of the body in relation to other parts as well as the rates of movements of the body parts. These are automatic functional process of human body.
- **Vestibular sense:** The movement of the fluid stimulates the firing of receptor neurons which then tells is also known as the vestibular sense **(Fig. 2.14)**.

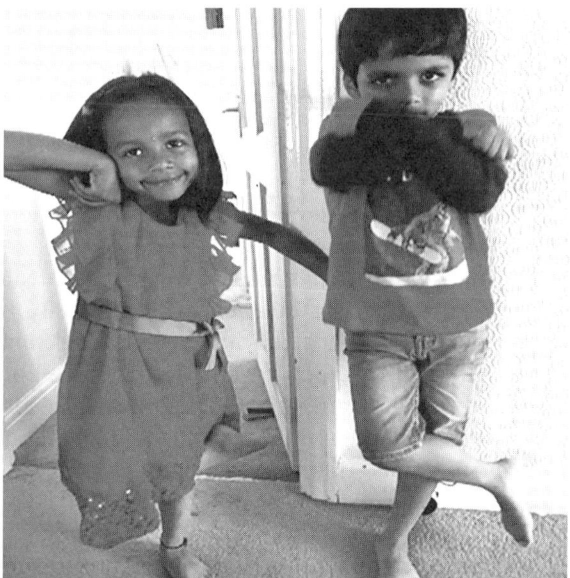

Fig. 2.14: The sense of balance

- **Extrasensory perceptions:** Extrasensory perceptions are defined as having awareness beyond the normal senses, such as vision or hearing and is what some people call the "sixth sense". Example—telepathy.

MUSCULAR AND GLANDULAR BEHAVIOR

The human body has two important systems in movement. In muscular system the functioning of skeletal system has greater role. It closely integrates in providing posture and movement to the various parts of body. The skeletal system protects the inner organs and transforms muscle contraction into locomotion. Our muscles are responsible for bodily movements, internal and external. The skeletal muscles enable the individuals to make movements by contracting and relaxing. The cardiac muscle is the muscle of heart and is responsible for pumping the blood.

The muscles and glands influence our behavior in many ways.

The muscle is a specialized tissue. It helps in excitement, contraction, and relaxation. The body movements like walking, running, balancing body postures, digestion, and elimination are important functions of muscular system. The movement of limbs, jaws, and tongue also occurring by movement of muscles. Muscles also help in communication functions such as speaking, writing, typing, gestures, and facial expressions.

Muscle Tone

Muscle tone is necessary for keeping the back and legs straight, the head held in an upright position and the abdomen from bulging.

Glands

There are two types of glands—duct glands and ductless glands.

Duct Glands

Duct glands releases the secretions of salivary, sweat, lacrimation, tears, etc. These are caused by emotions of sorrowfulness and pain. The imbalance of emotions causes indigestion and ulcers.

Endocrine Glands (Ductless Glands)

The endocrine glands secrete products called hormones which are chemical messengers that deliver stimulatory or inhibitory signals to the target cells.

The normal functioning of these hormones helps to healthy personality development. The irregularity of these secretions affect general metabolism, abnormality in human behavior.

- **Pituitary gland:** This is called the master gland, it secretes thyrotropin, a thyroid stimulating hormone. It helps in control of metabolism and balance the body temperature. The hyperactivity of this gland leads to gigantism and under activity leads to dwarfism.
- **Thyroid gland:** It is the largest gland in the body. The thyroid gland produces hormones called thyroxin. The normal secretion of thyroxin regulates oxygen levels in body. Hyperthyroidism causes nervous tension, insomnia, etc. Hypothyroidism causes forgetfulness, dullness, etc.
- **Parathyroid gland:** In human body four parathyroid glands located in the back side of the thyroid gland. Each lobe of thyroid has one pair of parathyroids. These glands secrete parathyroid hormone. These help in circulation of fluids. It plays an active role in balance of calcium. It promotes the activation of vitamin D into the active form.

Hyperactivity results in lack of interest, physical weakness, and softness of bones due to lack of calcium, and lethargy due nervous weakness.

- **Adrenal glands:** Adrenal gland stimulates secretion of cortisol, which plays a role in response to stress. The low secretions lead to mood disorders, depression, lack of interest in sexual activities, irritability, and fatigue. Oversecretion results in overexcitability, activeness, appearance of premature sexual characteristics, etc. Excess secretion in women leads to appearance of masculine characteristics such as moustache, hard voice, rough skin, and growth of hairs on the chest.
- **Gonads:** The gonads are sex glands and consist of the ovaries in females and testes in males. The sex hormones in males are called androgens and in females they are called estrogens and progesterone. These are important in development of personality traits and sexual interest. The irregular secretions of these hormones effects on maturation and changes in behavior in human personalities.
- **Pancreas:** Pancreas is both exocrine and endocrine function. It is an enlarged organ located posterior to the stomach. Glucose is secreted in response to hypoglycemia. Its action is mainly on the live cells. This increases the sugar level in blood. The hormone decreases uptake of glucose and its utilization of cells. Insulin regulates the normal glucose level in the blood. The increase of insulin leads to giddiness, sweating, unconscious, and weakness.
- **Pineal gland:** The pineal gland secretes a hormone called melatonin. It helps in maintaining the normal rhythms of sleep wake cycle, body temperature, etc. The melatonin influences metabolism, pigmentation, and menstrual cycle.

Thymus gland secretes the hormones which have a bearing on sex organs and sexual activities.

The knowledge of these glands and their functions help nurses to understand various signs and symptoms of diseases and the behavioral deviations associated with the activities among individuals.

NATURE OF BEHAVIOR OF THE ORGANISM

The behavior is controlled by physical and psychological process of mind and body. The behavior is elicited by a stimulus known as a response. Behavior has cognitive, affective, and conative components. The process or result of unification of these components into a whole is called integrated response.

INTEGRATED RESPONSE

The sensory organs are more prominent inputs to convert nerve signals in transmitting to brain. The receptors help in memory, attention and other cognitive processes. It is based on sensory input. This is integration.

The integration in nervous system responds in sending signals to muscles and regulations of hormonal secretion. The major two systems are sending signals to the body muscles, glands and organs. One is nervous system and the other is endocrine system.

The ability of learning, thinking, remembering possible by integration. The non-coordination receptors and effectors leads to physical mental disorders in human behavior.

Integrated response is the process of bringing simple reflexes and motions into more sophisticated responses.

CONCLUSION

The nurse should understand the interrelationship between the body and mind. The nurse helps to alter the behavior of patient by understanding body mind relationship in diagnose the disease. The knowledge on influence of genetics and behavior helps nurse in understanding the causes of major health problems in human being.

QUESTIONS

Essay Questions

1. Explain body-mind relationship behavior in detail.
2. Explain the role of nervous system in behavior.
3. Describe the role of muscles and glands on the individual behavior.
4. What behavioral effects are produced by endocrine glands? Explain.
5. Explain the effect of heredity and environment on human behavior.

Short Notes

1. What are the levels of consciousness?
2. Explain the concept of "Nature versus Nurture".
3. Explain in detail psychology of sensation.
4. Endocrine glands.
5. Describe the relationship between genetics and behavior.

Brief Questions

1. Define neuron.
2. Function of pituitary gland.
3. Abnormalities in genetics.

Fill in the Blanks

1. The basic unit of nervous system is ________________. (Neuron)
2. The nervous system consists brain and ________________. (Spinal cord)
3. The abnormalities of behavior caused by physical and mental ________________. (Disorders).
4. Hypnosis helps in ________________ of behavior. (Modification).
5. The word genetics is derived from the Greek word ________________ means beginning. (genetics)

Multiple Choice Questions

1. The basic unit of nervous system is ....
   a. Skin
   b. Neuron
   c. Hair
2. Endocrine glands are .... glands.
   a. Ductless
   b. Duct
   c. Synapse

3. Alzheimer's disease affects
   a. Vision
   b. Touch
   c. Memory
4. The right hemisphere controls movement and receives information from the .... side of the body.
   a. Left
   b. Right
   c. Back

Answers

1. b	2. a	3. c	4. a

3 CHAPTER

Cognitive Processes

Learning Objectives

- **Attention:** Types of attention, duration and degree, alterations
- **Perception:** Meaning, principles, factors affecting, errors
- **Learning:** Nature, type, learner and learning, factors influencing, laws and theories, process, transfer, study habits
- **Memory:** Meaning, type, nature factors influencing, development theories and methods of memorising and forgetting
- **Thinking:** Type and levels, stages of development, relationship with language and communication
- **Intelligence:** Meaning, classification, uses, theories
- **Aptitude:** Concept, types, individual differences and variability
    - Psychometric assessment of cognitive processes

INTRODUCTION

Cognitive comes from the Latin word "Cognito" meaning to apprehend or understand.

Cognition is the process of acquiring knowledge through our thoughts, experience, and senses. The process of thinking, perception, and memory are studied in the branch of cognitive psychology. In philosophical view, the subject psychology is rationalized by strengthening cognitive processes. The subjects of philosophy, neuroscience, and linguistics are related to cognitive science. In cognitive process, the mind is largely identified with the brain and working as organism in development of personality traits. The sensory areas of the brain produce consciousness of stimulus in creation of new ideas.

The definition of cognitive process is the performance of a cognitive way or process in movement that affects the mental contents. Psychology refers to the performance of some composite cognitive activity or an operation that affects mental processes. These are possible by process of thinking and remembering. Cognitive process is known as thought process. It covers the thoughts of behavior, perception, information storage, retrieval, and abstract processing. It is used in creativity by existing knowledge of human being. The ability to acquire knowledge and skills of cognition is influenced by social and psychological conditions of human environment. In psychology, the cognitive processes such as attention, perception, learning, memory, intelligence, and thinking are very important in human behavior **(Fig. 3.1)**.

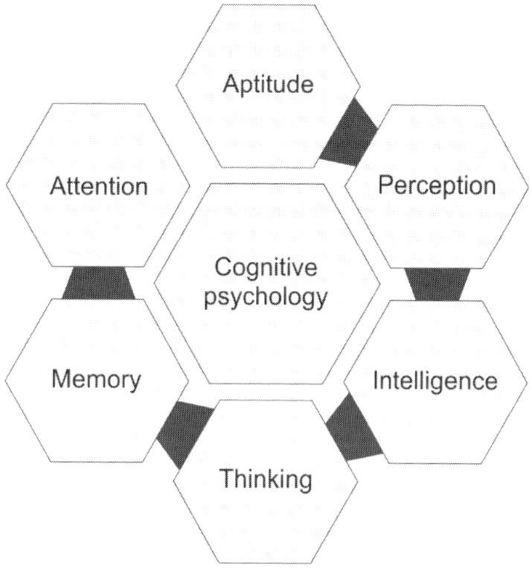

Fig. 3.1: Areas of cognitive processes

AREAS OF COGNITIVE PROCESSES

- **Attention:** The activity concentrating on a particular matter is called attention. Attention is an important characteristic in conscious of mind to acquire knowledge. It is an idea at a particular time, to the exclusion of other objects or ideas.
- **Perception:** The interpretation of sensory stimulus reaching to sense organs and brain is known as perception. It is a meaningful process of organizing and integrating stimulus.
- **Memory:** Memory is another important cognitive ability in decision-making by previous experience. The power to store experiences and to bring them into the field of consciousness sometimes after the experience has occurred is called memory. Studying human memory is a large part of cognitive psychology.
- **Thinking:** Thinking is also important cognitive activity in the form of information processing. It is a goal-oriented behavior of mental process by analyzation with ability of reasoning.
- **Intelligence:** Intelligence is the way to achieve goal with different kinds of reasoning, perception, memory, and attention processes.
- **Aptitude:** Aptitude means the ability or a particular skill or a potential. It is a special ability.

ATTENTION

Types of Attention, Duration and Degree, Alterations

Attention is the focus of consciousness on a particular object or idea at a particular time and away from other thoughts. Our attention is affected and distributed among the stimuli around us.

The changing levels of attention depend on size, color, novelty, and sound in surroundings. It is a very important cognitive process in human behavior. Attention is the cognitive process focused on a particular object.

Attention process is in two varieties. One is in selecting from external process of sound, images, and smell. Another is in selection from internal process of thoughts to get consciousness.

Attention is a complex cognitive function which is essential in every moment of human behavior. It is also depending on observational process.

The process of attention starts by observation. It involves with two mental activities. They are attention and perception. The observational process in attention followed by special attention is called perception. It gives clarity on decision-making. Thus, attention is not merely a cognitive process but also it is essential in determination by emotions, interest, attitude, and memory.

Definitions

Dumville: Attention is the concentration of consciousness upon one object rather than upon another.

Ross: Attention is the process of getting an object or thought clearly before the mind.

Morgan: Attention is being keenly alive to some specific factors in our environment. It is preparatory adjustment for response.

Types of Attention

- Voluntary attention or volitional attention
- Involuntary attention or non-volitional attention

Voluntary Attention or Volitional Attention

Voluntary attention occurs by necessity and automatically receives focus on conscious process. We need some conscious efforts in attainment of this process. The student is serious in writing answers to the questions in the examination hall. For example, Entrance **(Fig. 3.2)**, sudden noise, etc.

Types of Voluntary or Volitional Attention

- **Implicit volitional attention:** For example, The boss concentrates on performance of task from an employee in office to reach target or need warning on performance.
- **Explicit volitional attention:** This attention is obtained by repetition of acts. The athletes struggle hard and get attention in success of getting a shield. They need strong efforts by practice or repetition in reaching the goal.

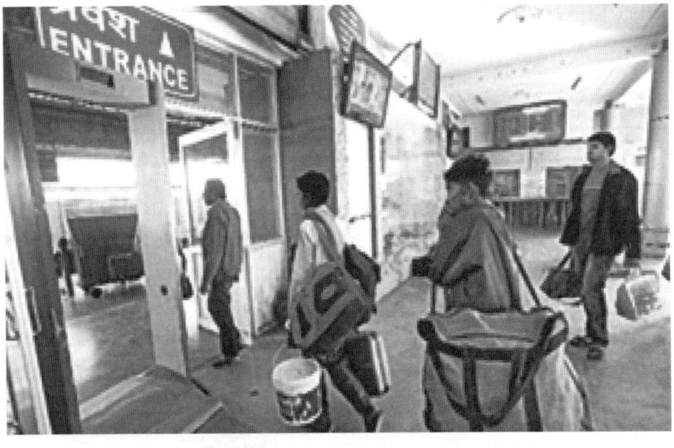

Fig. 3.2: Voluntary attention

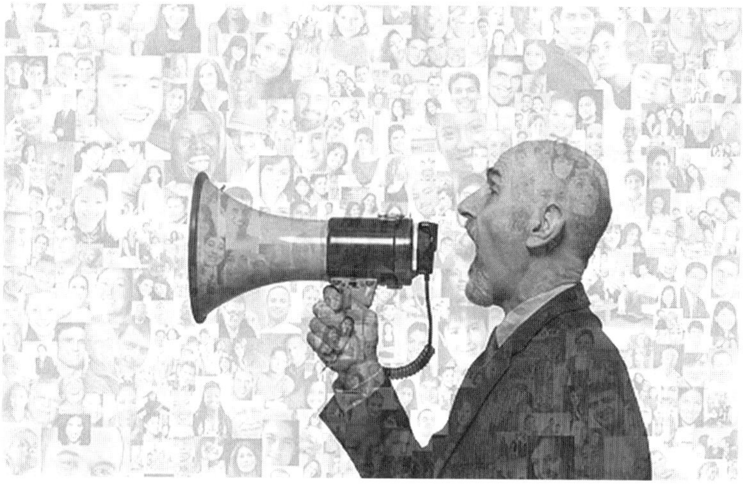

Fig. 3.3: Process of involuntary attention

Involuntary Attention or Non-volitional Attention

We cannot ignore the stimulus because of its intensity. It occurs spontaneously with our efforts. Most of the mother's attention is on her baby's crying voice, e.g., loud sounds **(Fig. 3.3)**, bright lights.

Factors Influencing Attention

People may focus on different objects from environment. But it is very difficult to attend a single object for a long duration. It is possible to keep conscious for a second or two on a single object. The duration of attention depends on the type of object, interest, etc. **(Fig. 3.4)**.

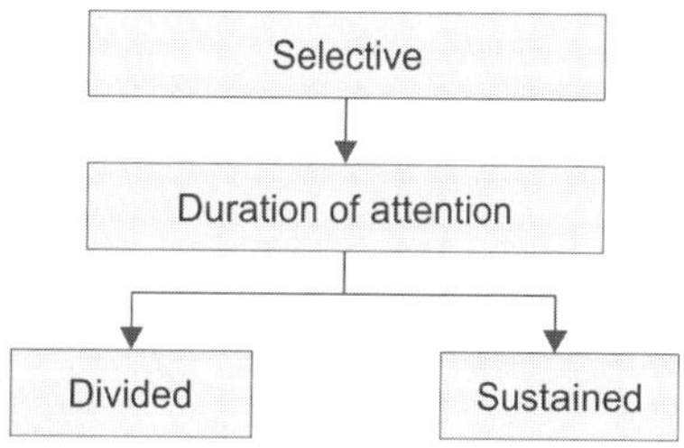

Fig. 3.4: Types in duration of attention

- **Selective attention:** It is also attention on moment of concentration on a particular aspect filtering from other aspects of surroundings **(Fig. 3.5)**.
- **Divided attention:** This type of attention is focused on two different aspects. It concentrates on two or more tasks simultaneously at a time. It means concentrating on more than one activity at a time **(Fig. 3.6)**.

  Psychologists say that focus is not strong by multiple objects. We cannot attend two things at a given time and there is possibility for division of attention. Attention rapidly shifts from one task to the other.
- **Sustained attention:** Both internal and external factors are important in sustained attention. Sustained attention is also commonly referred to one's attention span. People can get better at sustained attention as they practice it **(Fig. 3.7)**.

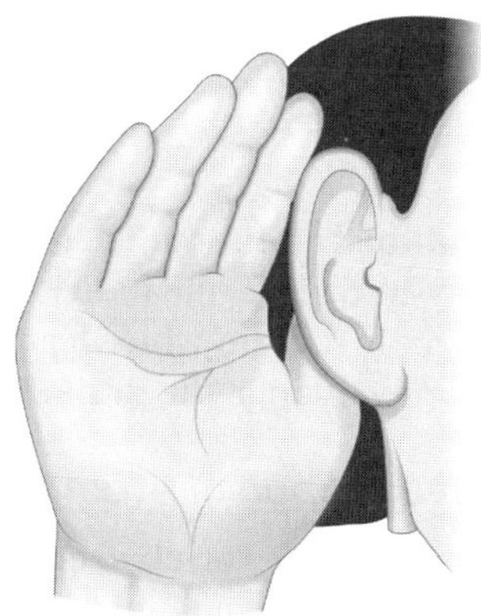

Fig. 3.5: Process of selective attention

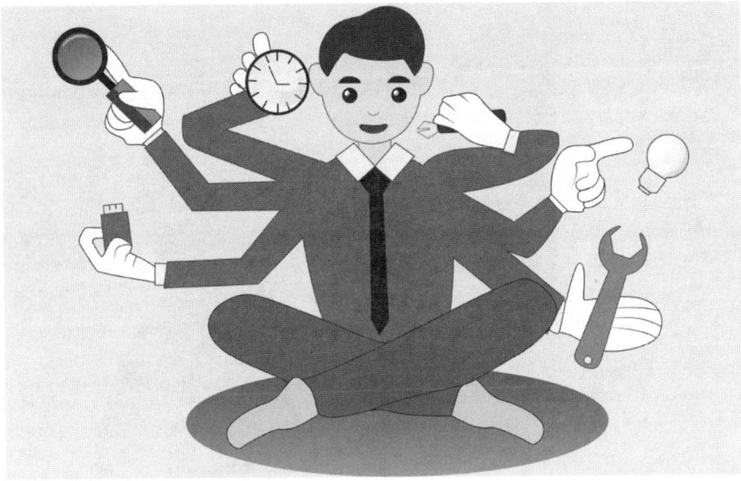

Fig. 3.6: Divided attention tasks

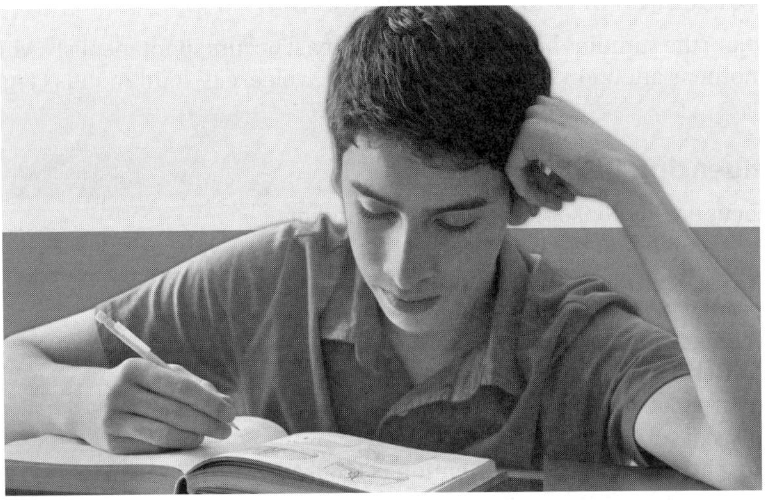

Fig. 3.7: Sustained attention task

- **Habitual attention:** There is no conscious effort or sensation in performance of activities. In day-to-day life, the individuals attend duties in habitual way. Sometimes the change takes place in routine, which leads to slow process. The frequency of change may become normal by repetition in the same style, e.g.: practice of driving and other learning skills.

Degree or Span of Attention

Attention focused on objects at a time is considered as degree of attention. It depends on factors of age, duration, and function of brain.

Span means the number of objects or events one individual can attend in a given time and at a glance, number of letters and digits one can see and reproduce.

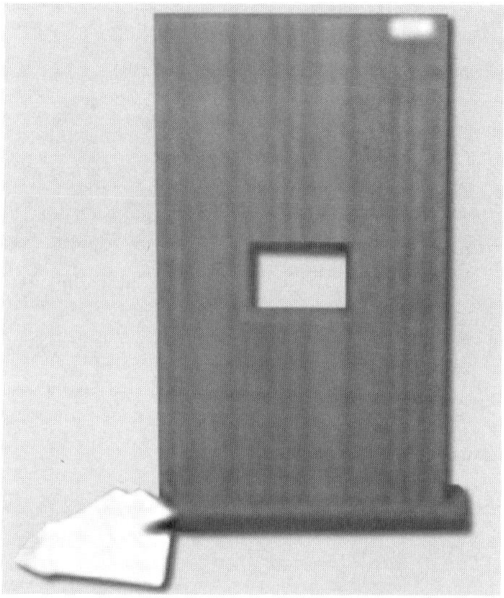

Fig. 3.8: Falling door tachistoscope

Tachistoscope **(Fig. 3.8)** is an apparatus designed to expose objects for a brief space of time. A subject is given a momentary glance from 1/5th to 1/10th of a second on regular or irregular groups of dots or letter and is required to tell how many he had observed.

The individual ability is evaluated by span of attention. The stimulus of attention on several objects proves the capability of individual performance. It may differ from one individual to another. The span of attention depends on size, color, distance, and duration in organizational process.

The psychologists proved that the normal span of attention is 7. Most of the cases have shown that the individual can focus nearly five digits or five letters in a single act of attention.

The attention focus may differ on kind of task, interest, age, and sense organs. Some children are short in span of attention due to malfunctioning of brain. The hyperactivity also leads to fluctuations in attention. Some distractions may disturb attentional process. It leads to irritation and distress.

Sir William Hamilton (1959) was the first to carry out the experimental study in this field. Later on, serial studies were carried out to reveal significant facts. Allerback (1929) studied the span of attention to test the number of dots, words, figures, colors, etc.

A falling door tachistoscope was used for the measurement of span of attention. Tachistoscope is an apparatus having a window in its middle portion that is called screen. The window is covered by an aluminum plate, which is connected with the lever. When the lever is pressed, the screen opens for 1/10 sec or 100 ms. In that short period, the subject reads the number of dots/alphabets and tells the same. Nine cards with black dots/alphabets (ranging from 3 to 11) were used. The dots/alphabets were made with black ink on white background. The size of the cards was 12 × 8 cm. The subject was provided a chair and the apparatus was placed on a stool in front of the subject so that the subject can easily see the dots in the window.

Distraction

"A distraction may be defined as any factor which normally tends to break up attention." **Prem Prakash.**

HR Bhatia: Distraction may be defined as any stimulus whose presence interferes with the process of attention or draws away attention from the object to which we wish to attend."

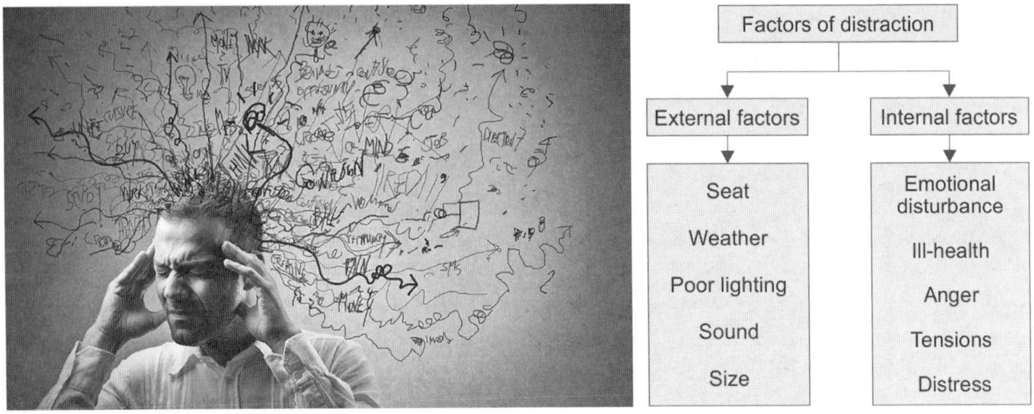

Fig. 3.9: Distracted person and sources of distraction

Sources of Distraction

- **External factors:** The distraction causes for poor performance in attention. They are irritating events **(Fig. 3.9)**, bad weather, poor lighting, irritating sounds, and discomfort seat which are the external factors of distractions of attention.
- **Internal factors:** Emotional disturbance, ill-health, anger, fear, tensions, lack of motivation, distress, and lack of interest are the internal sources of distraction of attention.

Determinants of Attention

The general conditions of attention depend on physical, emotional, and mental process of mind.

- **Nature and stimulus:** The size of object and color focus mind to get attention. The attraction depends on variety in size, beauty, etc., e.g., the pretty child, nature of climate, and comfort of seating are effective stimulus to capture attention.
- **Intensity of attention:** Good music, smell of favorable dishes, and contrast lighting turns mind to stimulate attention. Special design of buildings also attracts mind to get attention of the individuals.
- **Quality:** Different varieties also attract our mind to focus to think on a particular object or process. The special sounds, contrast of colors, and difference in taste may divert our attention.
- **Repetition of stimulus:** The repetition is one of the factors in improving our attention. The repeated songs and words may lead to special attention.
- **Movement of the stimulus:** The moving stimulus catches our attention than the other stimulus. The scrolling in television and changing colors may catch our attention. The business group may use different techniques by this type of attention.
- **Novelty:** Novelty means newness. The variety is an important attention to create interest toward new items. The sales people choose a variety of methods to improve sales in their business. The demo of the new product, sample attracts public to buy the new product.

Internal Determinants

Internal factors: The internal sources are very important in process of attention. These factors depend on our interest and attitude in performance.

Interest

The interest is most essential in focus of attention. Our attention captures on observation toward a particular point to continue the process of information, for example, watching a movie of a favorite hero or heroine or musician or director helps to focus attention and creates anxiety to watch a particular film. We pay more attention by interest.

- **Motives:** The motives or drives are important in process of attention. The motives of hunger and thirst are very curious in fulfilling their desires.
- **Anxiety:** It is one of the internal determinants of attention. The students are very anxious to read questions while writing examination and eagerly wait to know the results. They may focus attention in comparing to their class mates. The business team is curious in comparing profits with others business team.
- **Moods and attitudes:** The good mood gives keen attention on special objects. The mood disorders disturb our attention and attitudes in goal setting. The decision-making is difficult with mood disorders. So it is also one of the internal determinants of attention.
- **Health factors affect attention:** The emotional and mental illness disturbs attention in different ways, lack of interest, fear, tension, etc. The discomfort may cause some more disorders of health. Poor diet, lack of rest, and lack of sleep **(Fig. 3.10)** disturb mind and lead to ill-health.

We may lose our attention by some of the distractions. Cognitive process of memory loss also depends on internal factor of attention. The receptors and effectors are very important in managing good health.

Visual problems and auditory problems cause improper process of attention.

The sociopsychological reasons also cause physical ill health. The utilization of resources like receiving stimulus and response may cause normal functioning of body.

Medical facilities, health awareness, toleration of failures, and learning abilities cause psychological well-being of human behavior.

The serious issues affect our health by traumatic brain injury, stroke, learning disabilities, visual disorders, dementia, anxiety, depression, and emotional trauma.

Good exercise, physical fitness, and other relaxations improve our concentration in responding to stimulus in process of attention.

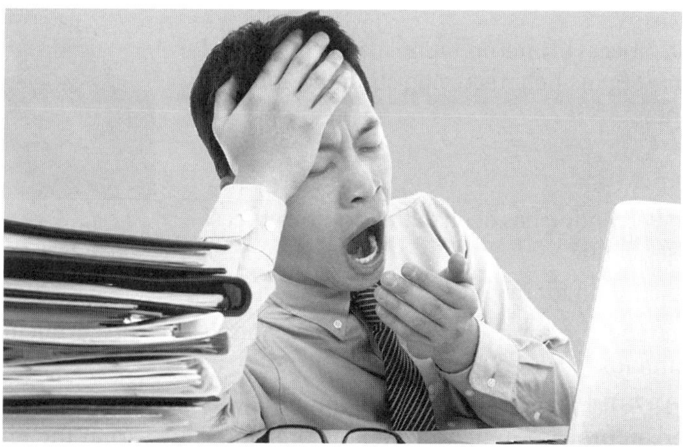

Fig. 3.10: Lack of sleep effects on health

PERCEPTION

The sense organs' role is very important in interpretation of stimulus. The sensations are transmitted to brain and nervous system. The mind and body relation is very important in receiving information from surroundings which has effects on behavior. The stimulus is influenced by all these interpretations. Previous experience and attitudes play major role in perceptual process of different objects in day-to-day life.

Sense of perception is the second step in observation. Perception gives meaning to sensation.

Perception = Sensation + Meaning

We sense qualities and perceive objects.

Sensation + Thought = Perception

In **Figure 3.11**, the process of perception leads to different thoughts. It is an optical illusion. It appears different to one individual from another. In one way, it appears as a young lady and in another as old lady or the child covered body with warm clothes and feather on head. There is no clarity on theme of the same figure. These expressions reveal that the information proceeds to the attitude of people in a particular moment.

Sensation is the process by which stimuli are detected, identified, and gauged. Sensation merely reveals information while perception is the interpretation of the information received.

The interpretation of stimulus is known as perception. The experience may give awareness in perceiving the objects.

The previous experience or guidance helps the child in identifying different animals, names of people perceived by guidance of parents, and elders learned from their childhood experiences.

Perception is a process of interpretation. It is an integrated process. The sense organs help receiving stimulus and give clarity in perception.

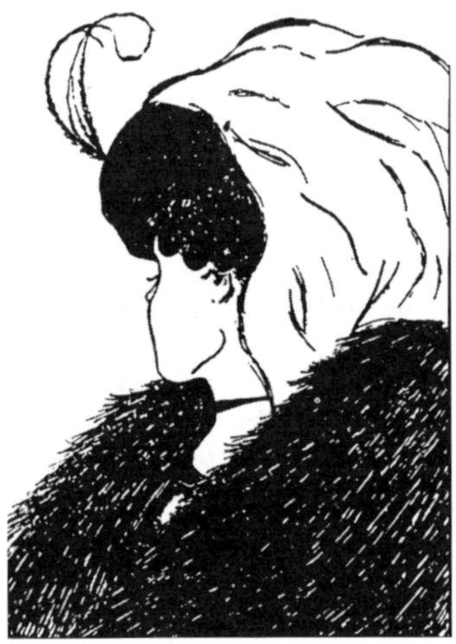

Fig. 3.11: The process of perception (optical illusion)

Definitions

(Forguds 1966): "Perception has been defined as the process of information extraction."

Hebb, 1966: "Preparation for responses."

EG Boring, HS Langfield, and HP Weld (1948): "Perception is the first event in the chain which leads from the stimulus to action."

RE Silverman (1976): Perception is an individual's awareness aspect of behavior, for it is the way each person processes the raw data he or she receives from the environment, into meaningful patterns.

William James, an American psychologist, has expressed that the appearance of the world may be different than watching it in a meaningful way.

In process of perception, individual concentrates on stimulus by common observation in proceeding of interpretation. In discrimination of stimulus, the visual interpretation may notice variations.

Gestalt psychology: Gestalt is a German word. Gestalt means seeing the whole picture all at once. This is explained by different principles of perception.

Principles of Perceptual Organization

Figure–ground Relationship

In this principle, following **Figures 3.12A and B** can be perceived more meaningful of a figure standing out from a back ground. For example, letters written with a white chalk piece are perceived clearly in the background of a blackboard.

In **Figures 3.12A and B**, two faces can be seen in the background of a white color. So, the white background can be perceived as a vessel in the background of two faces.

Grouping of Stimuli in Perceptual Organization

According to the Gestalt principle, the objects can be perceived with different meanings being as whole or dividing into parts. Gestalt gave priority to the whole than part in perceptual process.

The lines most closely resemble each other are perceived as units. In **Figure 3.13,** it is four horizontal lines or three items.

Proximity

Proximity means nearness. The objects which are nearer to one other may be perceived as circle while in separation.

The five circles in **Figure 3.14** are placed without proximity. The circles are given meaning grouped in another circle **(Fig. 3.15)** is knowns as Perceptual organisation in proximity.

Similarity

Stimuli need not be nearer to each other for perception. In **Figure 3.16**, we perceive stars and circle separately.

The example above appears as single unit because all the shapes have similarity.

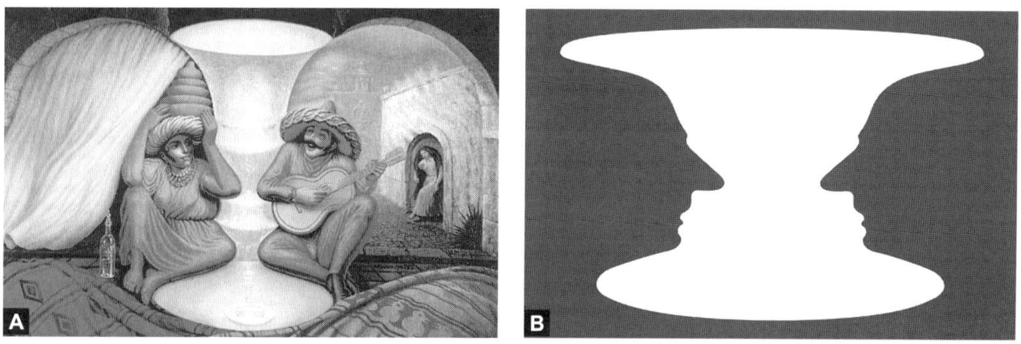

Figs. 3.12A and B: (A) Reversible configuration; (B) Vase face stimulus

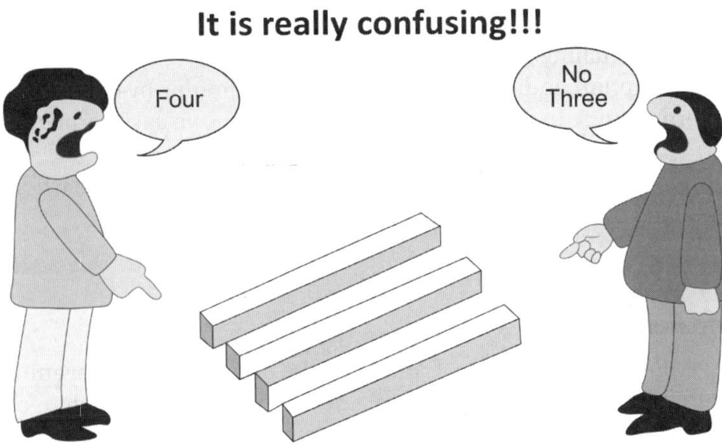

Fig. 3.13: Grouping of stimuli in perceptual organization

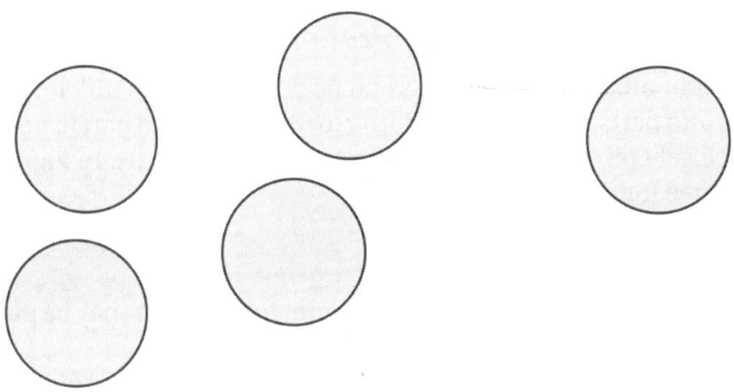

Fig. 3.14: Perceptual organization without proximity

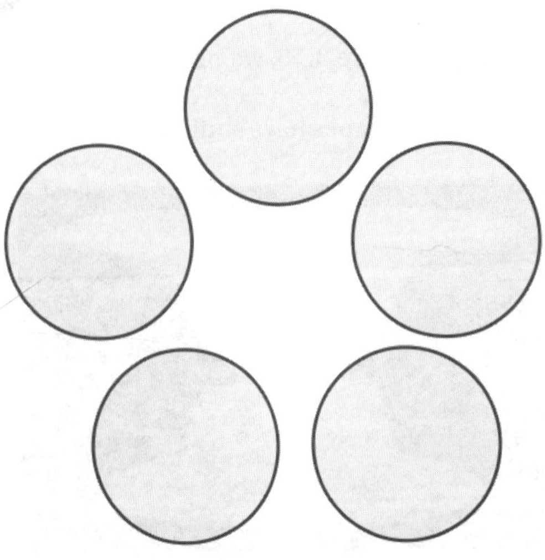

Fig. 3.15: Perceptual organization in proximity

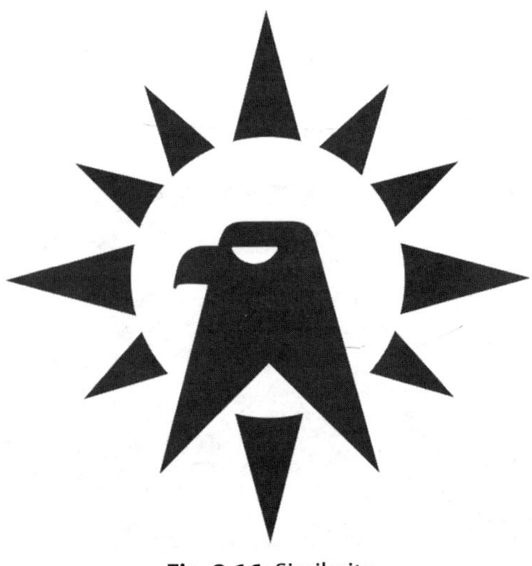

Fig. 3.16: Similarity

Continuity

Any stimulus which extends in the same direction **(Fig. 3.17B)** or shape will be perceived as a whole which may appear as another shape in continuity.

Naturally the viewer's eye catches that in full figure than part in this perceptual process **(Figs. 3.17A and B)**.

Closure

When a stimulus is presented with gaps, the human tendency is to perceive that **(Fig. 3.18)** as complete one by filling the gaps psychologically.

In **Figure 3.18**, rectangular shaped lines with gaps psychologically give a meaning of one particular shape. We are perceiving those four lines in a meaningful way as a rectangle.

Symmetry

Objects which are having symmetrical shape are perceived as groups. This is giving symmetry in perception **(Fig. 3.19)**.

Perceptual Constancy

Factors of Instability in Perceiving

- Size constancy
- Brightness or color constancy
- Perception of depth
- Visual monocular cues

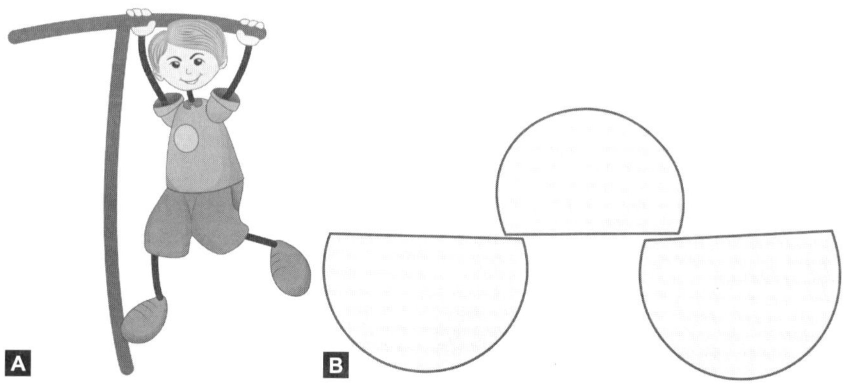

Figs. 3.17A and B: Continuity

Fig. 3.18: Closure

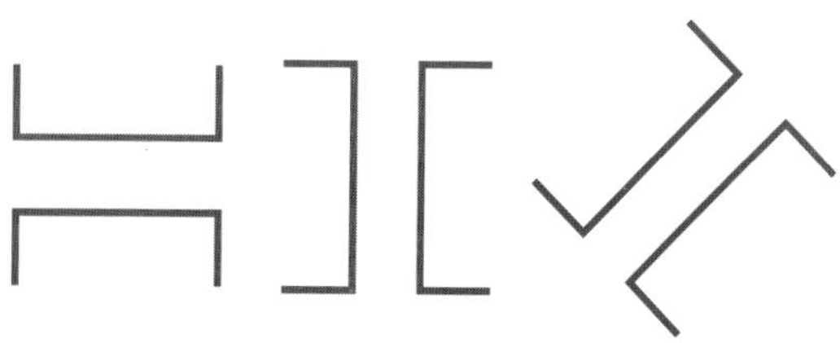

Fig. 3.19: Symmetry

The person's height and size appear small in size from top of the building. The object is stable but instability in perceiving the same due to gap in distance.

Perceptual constancy depends upon several factors like past experience, habits, motivations, thinking, learning, imagination, etc.

Types of Perceptual Constancy

There are different types of perceptual constancies. They are shape and size, brightness and color, size constancy, etc.

Depth Perception

Ability of a person to perceive the distance is known as depth perception. The judgment in perception depends on intelligence, grasping, and remembering in receiving stimulus by interpretation. This is very important ability to judge the distance between objects and perceiving stimulus. For example, passengers traveling by bus may perceive that the trees or pole are moving instead of the movement of their vehicles.

Depth perception is the ability to perceive space and distance accurately. It is also known as third dimension. In **Figures 3.20A and B,** we may perceive that most of the vehicles are moving on a busy road.

Cues: Cues are certain signs that are useful in decision-making by imagination of exact size or shape in dimensions. Cues are of two types:

1. **Binocular cues:** Cues which help in the perception of depth by integrating the images, symmetry with both eyes are called binocular cues.
   - **Convergence or divergence of eyeballs:** When the object moves nearer and nearer to our eyes, our eyeballs converge, and as the object moves away from us, the eyeballs diverge. This process acts as a binocular cue to perceive the depth. In **Figure 3.21**, the near objects appear clearer than the distant objects. For example, in **Figure 3.21**, a hill in far of distance appears farther away because the details do not seem clearly.
2. **Monocular cues:** These are the cues that can operate when only one eye is looking. Some of such cues are as follows:

   In **Figure 3.21**, the room is covered with several glass cues in different dimensions. It sets in similar dimensions. The distance separating the images and objects in appearance is small in size.

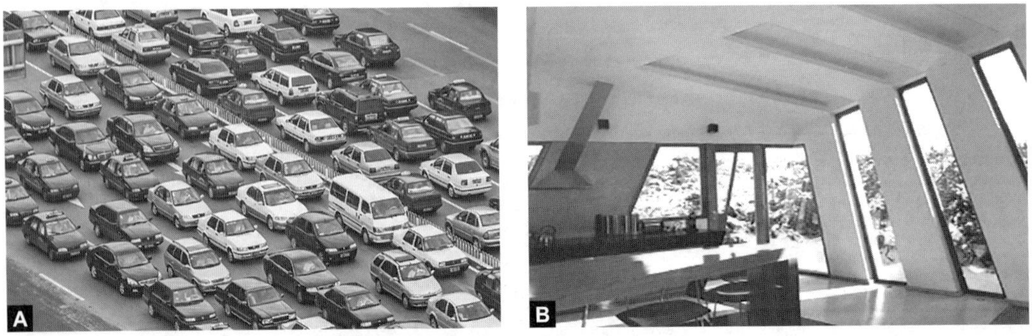

Figs. 3.20A and B: Depth in perception

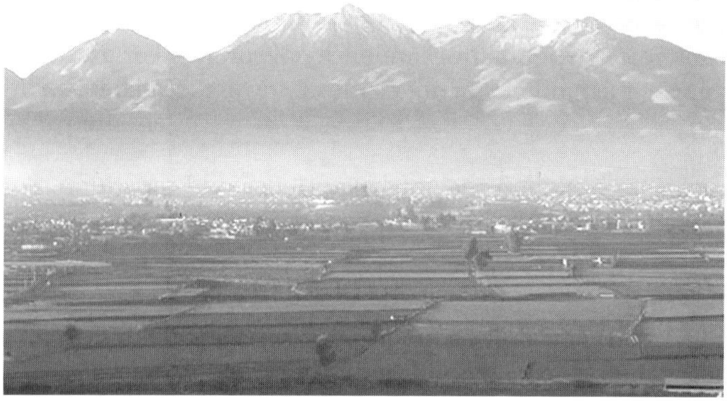

Fig. 3.21: Hill appears nearer

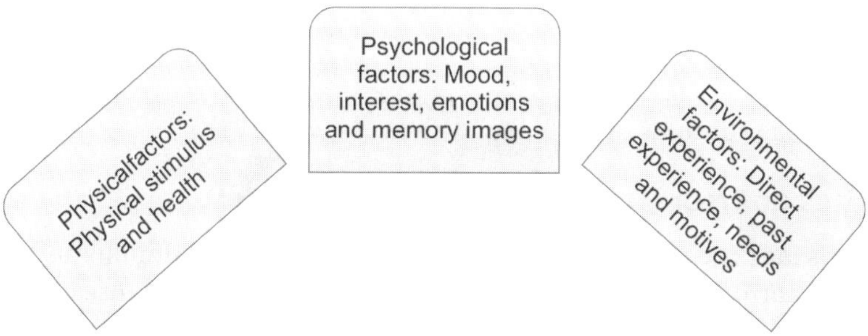

Fig. 3.22: Factors affecting perception

The Factors Affecting the Perceptions (Fig. 3.22)

Physical Factors

It depends on physical stimulus and health. There are individual differences in perceptual abilities. Two people may perceive the same stimulus differently.

The sensations increase constantly in every moment. The person who has illness cannot perceive perfectly and increases anxiety levels and psychological disturbance.

Psychological Factors

Mood, interest, emotions, and memory images.

Mood

The mood is depending on present circumstances of an individual engaged both physically and psychologically in mind.

Interest

Our acquired interest is also determining the object or objects that we perceive, e.g., the special attention will be given by the subject to reach their goal in time. The passengers waiting in a railway station may hear the sound of train and arrival on platform.

Emotions

Emotions are feelings in human behavior. Day-to-day life experience makes to identify voice of people without seeing the faces. The perception of these sounds' identity depends on previous experiences of their voice of popular or familiarity of sounds. For example, recognizing the voice of popular singer, the mother can notice the crying of their baby.

Memory Images

The memory images are based on previous experience and repetition. For example, blind people identify the people by their voice or by sound of their footsteps.

Environmental Process

Direct Experience

Direct observation helps for stimulus conformation.

Past Experience

The individual's past experience helps in development of mindset, attitude, sympathy, love and affection, and other personality traits.

Need and Motives

The aim is perceiving stimulus to fulfill their drives.

Abnormalities or Errors in Perception

The perception is the process of analyzation and discrimination of stimulus and interpretation. These are called as errors in perception. It may be due to defect in our sense organs or defective functioning of the brain. Several times, the prejudices in the individual, time of perception, unfavorable background, lack of clarity of stimulus, confusion, and conflict in mind are the factors for errors in perception.

There are two kinds of errors in perception (Fig. 3.23):

1. Illusion (Fig. 3.24)

Illusion is false in perception. For example, a rope appears as a snake in darkness. The voice of an unknown person is mistaken as a friend's voice. A person standing at a distance who is not known may be perceived as a known person.

Most of our illusions are visual and auditory.

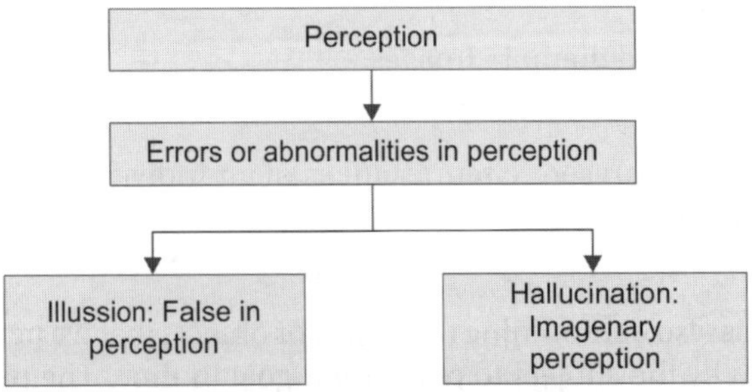

Fig. 3.23: Errors in perception

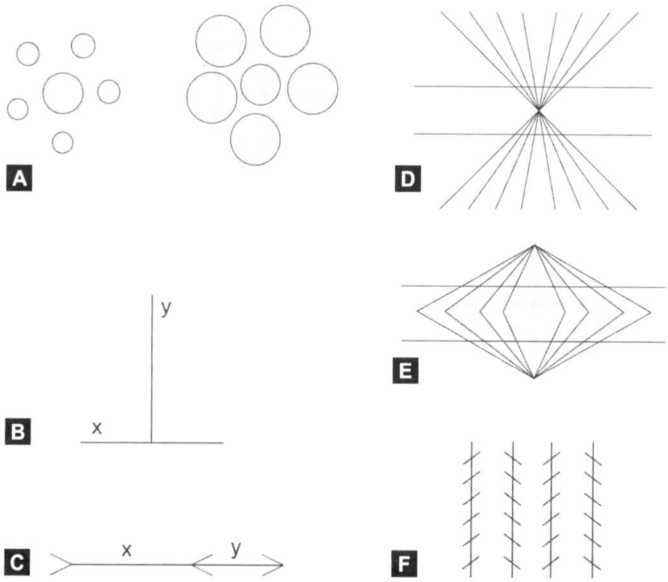

Figs. 3.24A to F: Examples of visual illusion. (A) Both the circles in the middle are same in size, but appear to vary; (B) Both horizontal and vertical lines are equal in length; (C) Both feather needed and arrow headed lines are equal in length: (D and E) The horizontal lines are straight: (F) The space between vertical lines, is equal

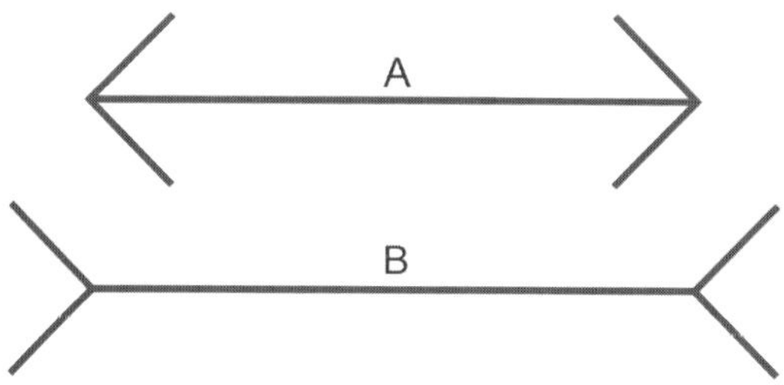

Figs. 3.25A and B: Error in perception- Illusion

Looking at **Figures 3.25A and B**, most of the people may say "B" looks long, simply because the points are facing in rather than out. But both lines are the same in length but arrows' direction makes us feel in wrong one is longer than the other.

Visual perception is the ability to see, organize, and interpret one's environment (**Figs. 3.26 and 3.27**).

2. Hallucination

Hallucination depends on psychological attention on a particular process which makes the individual appears the presence of objects.

The types of hallucinations are visual, auditory, and kinesthetic; when a person hallucinates, he hears, looks, and feels the nonexistent objects of stimuli.

Hallucinations are also common in people. It depends on psychological and emotional thought of the individual shown in **Figure 3.28**.

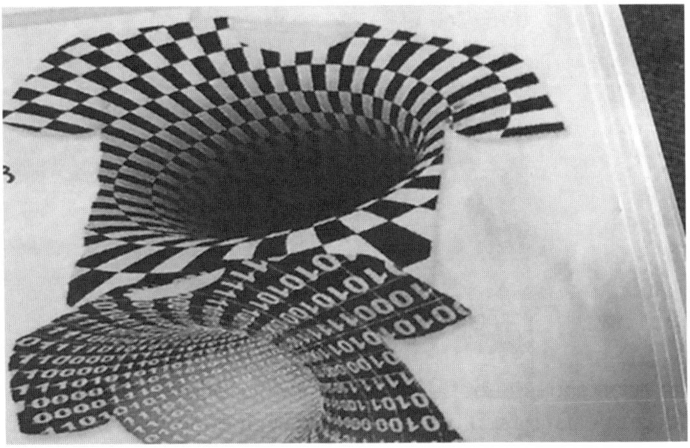

Fig. 3.26: Visual illusion in perception

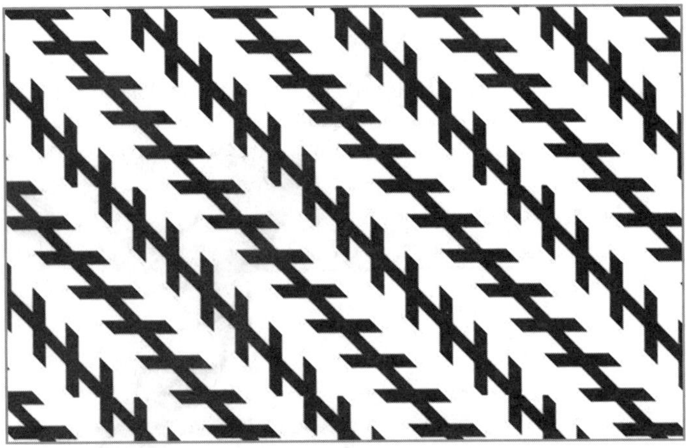

Fig. 3.27: Müller-Lyre illusion

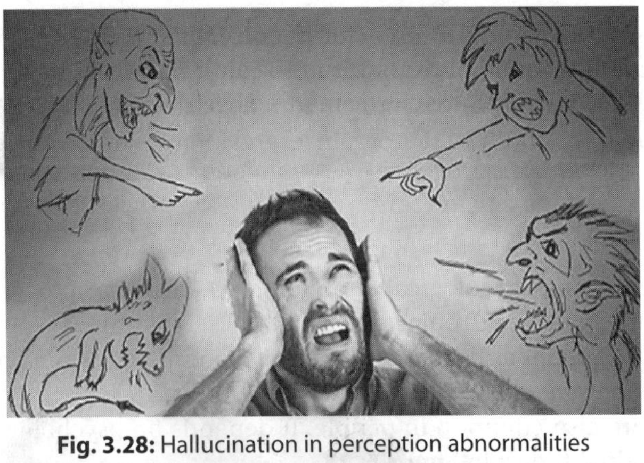

Fig. 3.28: Hallucination in perception abnormalities
Source: www.shutterstock.com

Extrasensory Perception (ESP)

Psychologists have named the perception that occurs without sensory stimulation as "extrasensory perception" (ESP). Some people can imagine future by their sixth sense. They can foresee the future with talent. This is also called as telepathy.

Parapsychology

Parapsychology is the study of paranormal psychic phenomena, including ESP. The scientific community rejects ESP due to the absence of an evidence base, the lack of a theory which would explain ESP, and the lack of experimental techniques which can provide reliably positive results; and considers ESP to be pseudoscience (Intelligence designing, Astrology).

Nursing Implication

Good and keen observational ability is an essential characteristic of a nurse. Observation involves attention and perception. The nurse should always concentrate on duties. Distraction of attention may lead to serious consequences of the death of a patient. Attention helps to understand the problems of patients. The follow-up programs may be implemented by the nurse to successful coordination between patient and nurse in periodical health check-up, etc.

LEARNING

Learning is a process of activity to gain knowledge, behavior, and skills. It is common in all human beings and animals. The perfectness in performance is possible by practice or repeated trials.

Example: Mother trains her child for breastfeeding. It is helpful to both mother and child. The child imitates parents in sitting, standing, walking, and speaking in childhood. The child learns many tasks in process of socialization. School atmosphere provides good guidance in social interaction and correction of behavior by teachers and parents in development of personality. It may be goal oriented and motivational process. Sometimes the learning occurs consciously or without consciousness. Learning also involves both physical and mental activities.

Definitions

Learning is defined as "any relatively permanent change in behavior that occurs because of practice and experience."

Woodworth (1945): "Any activity can be called learning so far as it develops the individual in any respect (good or bad) and makes him alter behavior and experiences different from what that would otherwise have been."

Henry P Smith: "Learning is the acquisition of new behavior or the strengthening or weakening of old behavior as the result of experience."

Kingsley and Gary (1957): "Learning is the process by which behavior (in the broader sense) is originated or changes practice or training."

Crow and Crow: "Learning is the acquisition of habits, knowledge, and attitudes. It involves new ways of doing things and it operates in individual's attempts to overcome obstacles or to adjust to new situations. It represents progressive changes in behavior. It enables him to satisfy interests to attain goals."

Gardner Murphy: "The term learning covers every modification in behavior to meet environmental requirements."

Nature of Learning

- **Learning is universal:** Learning is natural in all living organisms. The animal follows another animal in changing directions while walking on road. The human being learns by imitation and observation in day-to-day activities of life.
- **Learning through experience:** Ability of learning depends on intelligence and patience in practice. It is measured by number or duration in learning. It differs from one individual to another. The experience helps to individual in performance of the same task even after a long period.
- **Learning is a guide:** In learning process, parents, teachers, friends, and state and religion have major role. They are social agencies in managing social interactions and motivate the people toward learning.
- **Learning is never ending process:** There is no end in process of learning. The usage of new technology and inventories makes the individual to learn. The benefits motivate to learn new path in every moment of life. Learning is common from birth till death.
- **Learning is an adjustment:** Learning is an adjustment of individuals by modification of behavior toward growth and development. They acquire knowledge in forming behavior by learning new techniques. The acceptance for learning toward new process depends on necessities of individuals.
- **Learning is more essential:** The progress of human behavior in improvement of economic status and social and psychological conditions depends on adjustment of individual toward new culture, adopting new methods. The results provide satisfaction in individuals by consequences of performance and management of critical situations.

Learner and Learning

The learner is serious to get guidance from an expert in his learning process. Quality of learning depends on selection of role models, parents, teachers, books, scientists, etc. These are naturally helpful or guide the learner as in process of learning. Learning is the process of acquiring new or modifying existing knowledge, behavior, skills, and values of preferences.

Process of Learning

- **Motor learning:** These are possible by muscular coordination. It is helping them to get psychological support in leading life to fulfill their desires.
- **Verbal learning:** The child is weak in speech in primary level but gets perfectness by observational process. The preference in communication and clarity in speech are possible by verbal learning.
- **Nonverbal learning:** The sentence completion, writing skills are called as nonverbal learning process.

Factors Affecting Learning

- **External factors:** Hereditary places an important role in performance of skills and creates motivation toward new forms of human process. Some are fast in learning, and some are slow in learning; it depends on different reasons like practice, environment, competition, intelligence, interest, age, etc.
- **Internal factors:** Internal factors such as attitude, interest, heredity, curiosity, and competition motivate the goal. Achievement of goal raises speed and interest in learning. Goals should be specific and clear before practice of learning.
- **Motivation:** It stimulates the individual toward performance in a successful way.
- **Interest:** It encourages an individual to forward the individual in task performance.
- **Attention:** Attention is also one of the important internal factors of learning. The focus of attention is essential in perfectness of learning process. The poor performance slows the learning practice. The concentration or focus of consciousness upon one object or an idea helps in fast learning. If effective learning should take place, attention is essential. Instructors must secure the attention of the student.
- **Fatigue:** The fatigue becomes a barrier in progress of learning process.
- **Aptitude:** Aptitude is a special ability. An aptitude may be considered a special ability or special capacity besides the general intellectual ability which helps an individual to acquire a required degree of proficiency or achievement in a specific field.
- **Attitude:** Attitude is a psychological and mental readiness. It has greater role in performance of tasks. It depends on cognitive ability of thinking in creational process of learning.
- **Emotional conditions:** Emotions are strong feelings. Positive stress levels are important in balancing emotions.
- **Guidance:** It is very important in adoption for learning methods, facilities, tools, and suggestions. It leads toward perfectness in learning. They can identify the defects and tackle the weak candidates by testing their skills by providing special guidance. The good teacher manages variety of students in motivation of discipline and success in their career.

Types and Theories of Learning (Fig. 3.29)

- Behavioral learning
- Cognitive learning
- Constructive learning

Behavioral learning is based on outside stimuli. It is associated with brain and intelligence.

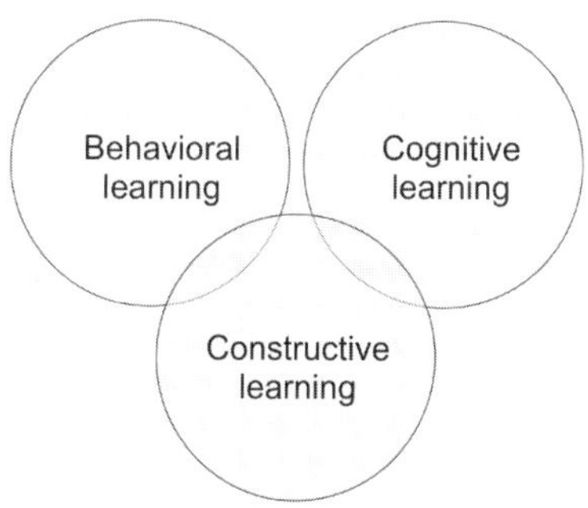

Fig. 3.29: Types of learning

Learning by Trial and Error

This theory was developed by Thorndike (1874–1949). Thorndike **(Fig. 3.30)** strongly believed that learning occurs by trial and error method. Thorndike explained through many theories that the individual tries to achieve perfectness by practice.

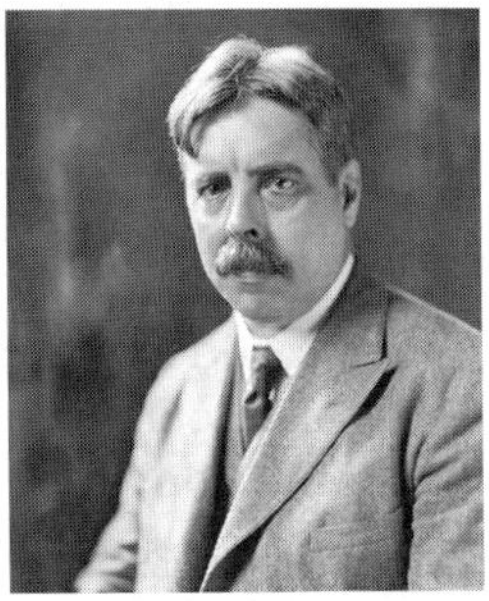

Fig. 3.30: EL Thorndike

Thorndike's experiment on cat in the puzzle is more famous among experiments on learning in psychology. The experiment is very simple. A hungry cat was inside the puzzle box and the dish filled with food was kept outside the box. The cat got temptation to eat food. It tried to catch food dish by jumping, pushing, and got irritated by failure in reaching goal. After several movements in puzzle box, the cat succeeded and pulled the string to open the puzzle box in a single attempt by experience in opening the door. It ate food happily. Thorndike gave chance to the cat to do the same task in different trails as task to repeat. The cat attempted trials to get food dish in short duration. Thorndike noticed that the repetition increases and errors decreased in completion of task. He concluded that cat learned to pull the string in opening puzzle box by desire of eating food. It is the connection between stimulus and response **(Fig. 3.31)**.

Thorndike studied the character of trial and error—using a box which he called "puzzle box."

In the beginning, the cat made several random movements like biting, clawing, dashing, etc.; gradually in subsequent trials, the cat reduced the incorrect responses (errors), as it could manipulate as soon as it was put in the box.

Thorndike conducted many experiments with maze and puzzle box learning in which cats and rats were used **(Fig. 3.32)**. He had demonstrated that through numerous trials and gradually improves his effort.

Most of the trainers follow these techniques for perfectness in preparation of champions in sports, games, and all fields of learning.

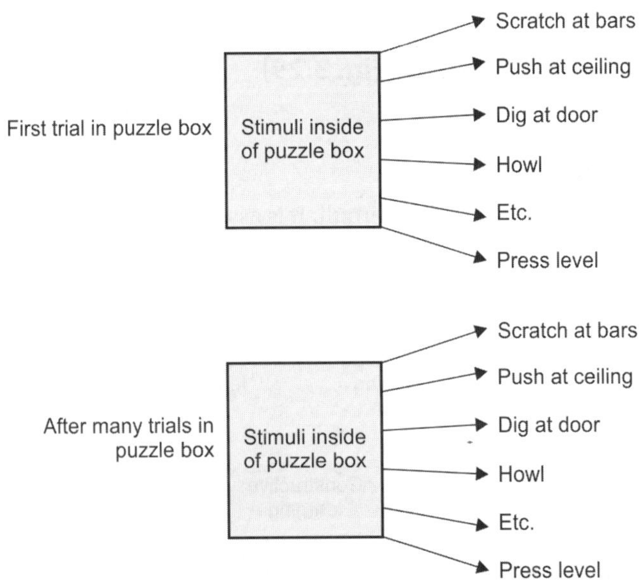

Fig. 3.31: Thorndike trial and error learning process

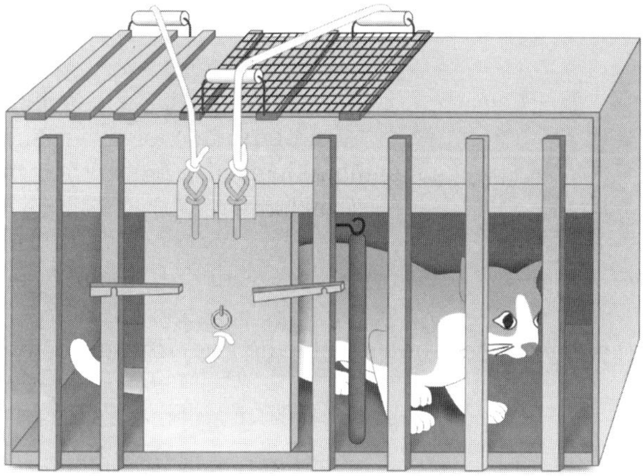

Fig. 3.32: Thorndike experiment on learning process

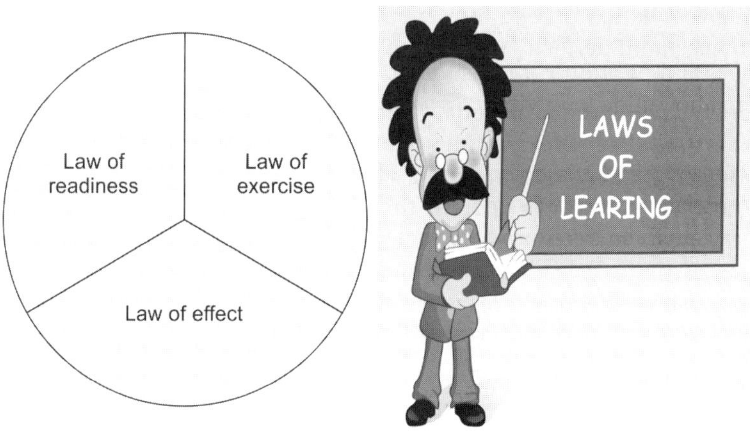

Fig. 3.33: Thorndike primary laws of learning

Laws of Learning

Thorndike Primary Laws (Fig. 3.33)

- **Law of readiness:** Learning is not possible without interest in topic. The physical and mental readiness is important in motivation for learning.

  This indicates that the animal or human being is motivated to learn. It gives pleasure and creates capability to tolerate pain even by delay in learning the process.
  - Goal
  - Interest
  - Toleration

  This law clearly shows that readiness of a person is very important in motivational process in learning.
- **Law of exercise:** This law is also known as law of frequency. The necessity or interest changes the attitude of person to continue the process by several exercises **(Fig. 3.34)** in

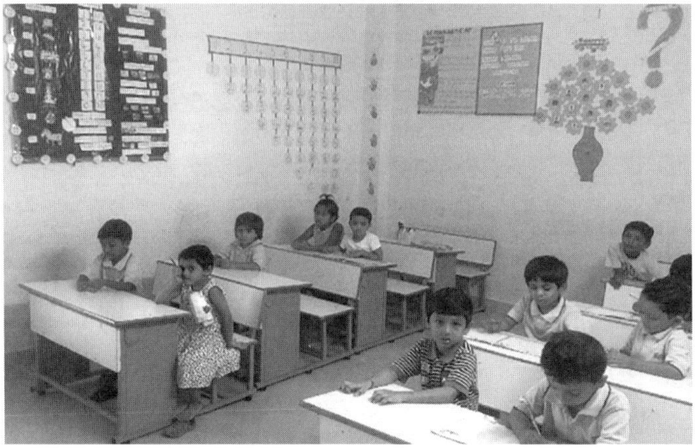

Fig. 3.34: Law of exercise and readiness

learning. It gives chance for long-term memory. This is also according to the statement that "practice makes man perfect." Most of the experts reached goal by trial and error process of learning.

- **Law of effect:** The learner will satisfy himself by repetition, memory in recollection of process. This strength creates confidence and pleasure toward the process of learning.

  By this, Thorndike meant that the probability of its occurrence is greater. In his experiment, if the hungry cat succeeded in opening the door, it would get its favorable dish to eat. The student feels pleasure in getting success in his education by repetition of tasks in class hours. The less exercise in tasks leads to failure in education, etc.

  This had a positive effect on its response. Rewards always strengthen connections between stimuli and responses, and on the other hand, punishment weakens connections.

The Law of Use and Disuse

- **Law of use:** It means that the person gets capacity of recollecting the learned process in short duration without more trials. It depends on confidence and effect of learning in previous.
- **Law of disuse:** It is decayed in memory and takes several trials to learn as in first attempt.

Secondary Laws

In addition to the three primary laws explained above, Thorndike has given five secondary or subsidiary laws also.

They are as follows:

- **Law of multiple response:** Confronted with new situations, the organism responds in a variety of ways before arriving at the correct response.
- **Law of attitude:** The zeal is important toward the progress in learning.
- **Law of associative shifting:** The subject may respond to the new situations and changes in stimulation in possible way called as associative learning process of shifting.
- **Law of prepotency of elements:** This law states that the learner is able to react in a selected way, by using his/her knowledge.

- **Law of response by analogy:** It means comparing a new situation to the previously learned one and thus giving a response by analogy.

As stated above, Thorndike formulated these laws on the basis of his experiments. According to the law of readiness, the cat was ready to learn, because it was hungry. This hunger motivated the cat to learn to open the door.

According to the second law, the cat was repeatedly given trials and exercise which strengthened its learning.

This encouraged the cat to continue its effort to learn to open the door. The secondary laws given by him support these findings. These laws are highly relevant to the field of education.

The Thorndike experiment proved that in many of our skills like, swimming, cycling, and riding, by repetition we will get perfectness. Teachers can make use of these laws in order to make their teaching more effective.

Learning Theory of Condition Reflexes

Psychologists conducted many experiments on animals and children before coming to certain definite conclusions which explain the process of learning. There are many theories in explanation of learning process of condition.

The term condition literally means "getting used" to, or "adjusted" to a new situation, or a stimulus. It is a process of substituting the original stimulus by a new one and connecting the response with it. It is an activity performed to obtain benefits under some conditions and restrictions without crossing the limits.

There are two types of conditioning theories:

Classical Conditioning

Ivan Pavlov, a Russian physiologist, 1849–1936, **(Fig. 3.35)**, who had already won the noble prize (1904), noticed that a dog began to salivate by food and decided to see whether a dog could be taught to associate food with other things, such as light or a tone.

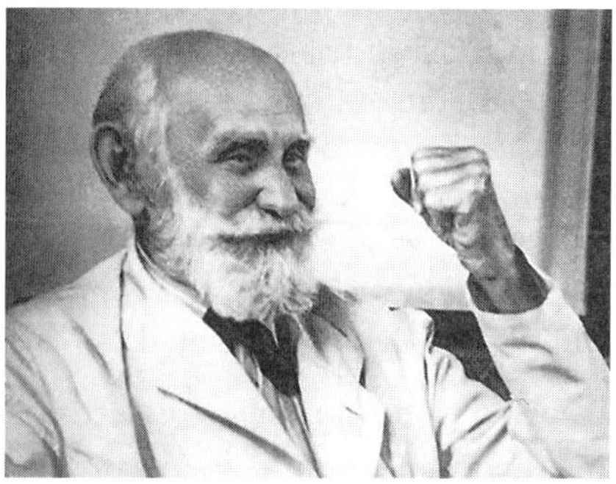

Fig. 3.35: Ivan P Pavlov

Pavlov designed an apparatus to measure the quantity of saliva produced in response to food (meat power). At the beginning of his experiment, Pavlov noted that no saliva flowed when he rang the bell. He then trained the dog by sounding the bell, and shortly afterward presenting food.

After the sound of the bell had been paired with food a few times, he tested the effects of the training by measuring the amount of saliva that flowed when he rang the bell and did not present food. He found that some saliva was produced in response to the sound of the bell alone **(Fig. 3.36)**. He then resumed the training-paired presentation of bell and food a few times and then tested again with the bell alone.

This theory states that CS (bell) becomes a substitute after pairing with UCS (food) and acquires the capacity to elicit a response. It is because the association (conditioning) is formed between CS and UCS.

Sub-principles of Classical Conditioning

There are certain sub-principles which explain the different phenomena of this experiment.

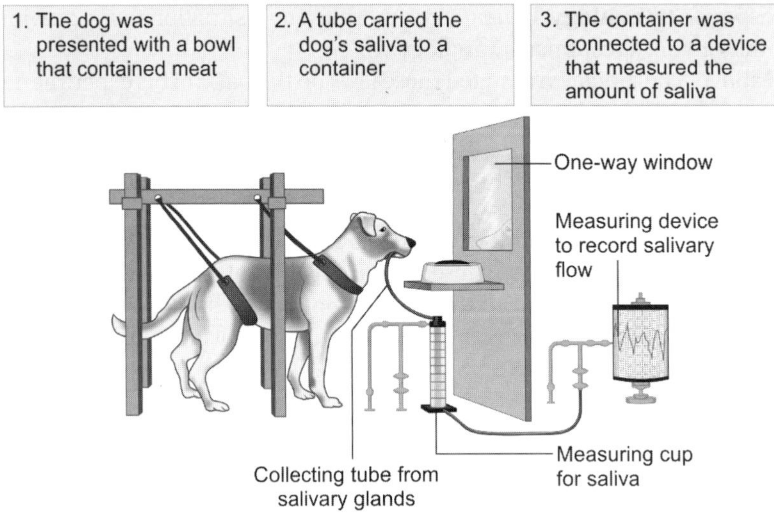

Fig. 3.36: Ivan Pavlov Classical conditioning experiment

Extinction and spontaneous recovery

Extinction means CS is presented alone without UCS for a number of trials, the strength of the CS gradually decreases. In this experiment, when only bell was presented without food for a number of trials, the dog stopped salivation gradually.

But when the CS (bell) was paired again with UCS (food) for some trials, the CR (salivation) recovered. This is known as "spontaneous recovery." In spontaneous recovery, the dog required less number of trials than the first time, because the association between CS and UCS still existed in the brain of the animal.

A tendency to respond to a stimulus which is similar to original one is called stimulus generalization; the greater the similarity, the more the generalization. In this experiment, the dog started salivating even before the sound of a buzzer which was similar to bell.

For example, if the dog is conditioned to salivate at the signal of red light, it will not salivate when green light is presented.

Operant Conditioning

In this theory, the learning process is based on condition using an instrument in fulfilling desire. Previously no idea of learning, the animal may touch an instrument getting some benefit, the animal planned to repeat the trials to get success. The organism's response depends on environment in achieving goal. This method of experiment was proved by American psychologist BF Skinner **(Fig. 3.37)**.

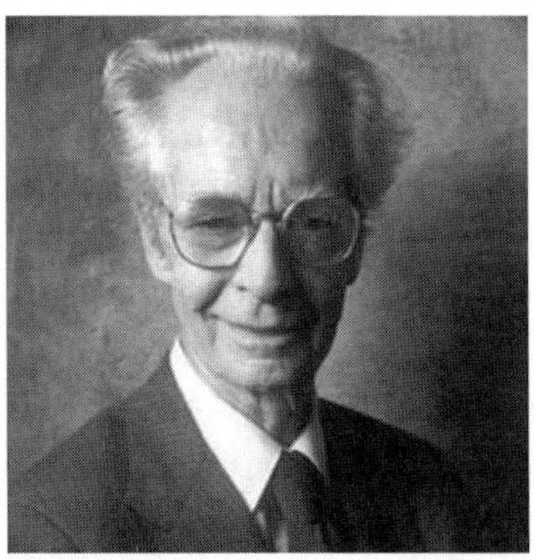

Fig. 3.37: BF Skinner

Skinner conducted his famous experiment by placing a hungry rat in a box called after his name "Skinner box" **(Fig. 3.38)**. It was arranged that the animal was free to move inside the box, but the pressing of the lever would get the animal a pallet of food in the tray as reinforcement. Arrangement was

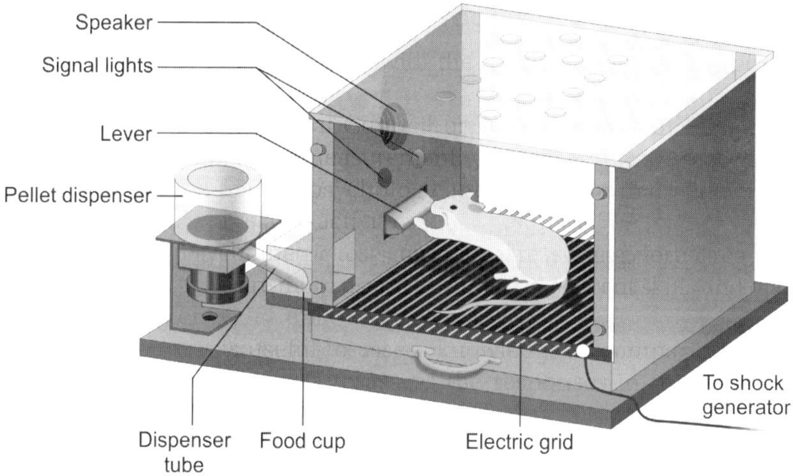

Fig. 3.38: BF Skinner experiment on operant conditioning

also made to record the number of pressings of the lever by a mechanical device. It was found in the beginning that the rat pressed the lever occasionally and used to get food as reinforcement for each pressing.

Gradually, as the animal learnt that the pressing of lever would give some food, it repeated the responses very rapidly. This rapid increase in pressing the lever is the indication of the animal conditioned to get food.

In day-to-day's life, most of the learning skills depend on reward to face the pain. Also, the reinforcement will be the motivating factor. It will make the organism to repeat its action.

Based on these experiments, Skinner made his famous statement "Rewarded behavior is repeated." Instrumental conditioning involves more activity by the learner than classical conditioning. Skinner conducted his experiments on different animals like pigeons, rats, etc.

Positive Reinforcement and Negative Reinforcement

Reinforcement is divided into two types:

1. Positive reinforcement
2. Negative reinforcement.

Reward is given for good in performance of task. These are useful in modification of behavior.

Operant conditioning is useful in shaping undesirable behavior and also in modification of behavior. Positive reinforcement like punishment is used to stop undesired responses or behaviors.

Operant conditioning is a term used to describe behavior which has been reinforced by reward or discouraged through punishment. A mother training the child by offering toys to learn cleaning of room, and schools encouraging the students by giving grades for neatness are some examples of positive reinforcement.

As a result, the girl's behavior (cleaning her room) has been modified (conditioned) because she has learned to associate a behavior with a reward.

The difference between operant and classical conditioning is that in classical conditioning, the conditional behavior (CR) is responded by stimulus.

Cognitive Learning

Learning by Insight

Insight means sudden thought. In day-to-day life, people face different incidents; some are interested in getting attention. It gives difficulty in reaching goal and motivates them to create ideas to get success without planning. Many times learning proceeds by more efficiency in achievement of goal. This is possible by understanding or perception of the situation.

Learning by perceiving the relationship in the scene and understanding situation is insightful learning. This theory was developed by a psychologist known as Wolfgang Kohler, who belonged to Gestalt School of Psychology.

According to Gestalt theory, perception of a situation as a "whole" gives better understanding than sum total of its parts. This theory tells that the situation in whole is better than viewed into parts.

Kohler conducted his most famous experiments on chimpanzee—called Sultan. In the experiment, Sultan was put in a cage and a banana was placed at some distance outside the cage. Then the chimpanzee was given two sticks, so constructed that one stick could be fit into another and made the stick longer.

The hungry Sultan **(Fig. 3.39)** first tried to catch bananas with hands and failed. Later it got idea to catch with single stick and not succeeded. Suddenly, Sultan got another idea to link both sticks, observed while playing and pulled the bananas.

While playing so, one of the sticks got fit into another and the stick became lengthier. This "sudden flash of idea" to reach food with longer stick was called "Insight," by Kohler. He concluded that the occurrence of insight to find solution to a problem is possible by perception of the whole situation. Kohler conducted many experiments on this line of learning to prove that just trial and error method is not enough to find solution for many complex problems.

Characteristics of Learning by Insight

- Insight is sudden thought.
- Insight develops usually after some failures in learning.

Insight is often used in problem-solving puzzles and riddles. It is also called as "**Aha experience**" or Archimedes "Eurekha."

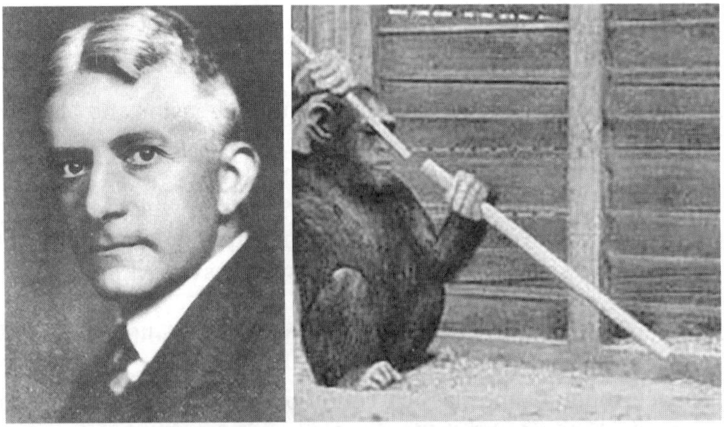

Fig. 3.39: Wolf gang Kohler Insight Leaning process

Trial and error is based on acquiring of knowledge, skills, interests, habits, and other personality characteristics. But it is absolutely insufficient for solving complex problems.

Insight occurs, when the individual sees in a flash, the solution to his problem or difficulty. It is not blind or stupid learning. The exercises discriminate ability in solving problems, and learning becomes a matter of insight rather than of trial and error.

Sign Learning—Tolman's Theory of Sign Learning

According to Tolman 1930, **(Fig. 3.40)**, learning takes place by cognition. The learner may feel easy to learn by some symbols, signs, digits, or figures. Example "O" (Zero) gives meaning of nil. "X" shows wrong, symbol for multiplication, letter in English alphabets, ?-Question mark, etc. The experience or repetition of the same figure or signs or symbols is good in recollecting thoughts in process of learning. The simple glance is faster in it than the other methods of learning. this theory called as sign learning theory.

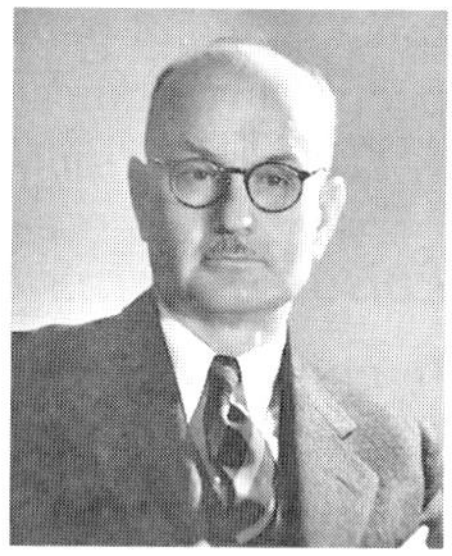

Fig. 3.40: Tolman

Tolman was well known for his experiments using rats and maze running **(Fig. 3.41)**. In a typical experiment by investigators in sign learning, a comparison was made between two groups of hungry rats in the maze. In these groups, each subject was given access to the maze without finding a food reward and little improvement occurred in time or error scores.

According to Tolman, the behavior depends on need system. This theory takes into consideration that learning is based upon some signs or clues leading to the goal. The organism learns not only the movement patterns but also the sign-significant relations.

Theory of Observational learning or Social Learning: Observational learning was first described by Albert Bandura. According to this theory, behavior observation influences the person in several ways. Most of the people learn by imitating people by their interest. Social interaction and social agencies have major role in this learning theory.

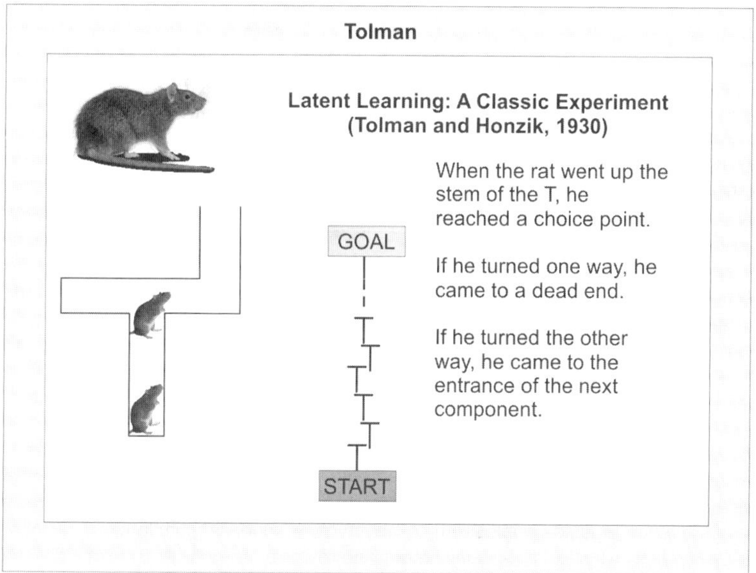

Fig. 3.41: Tolman's cognitive learning theory

Bandura's social learning theory explains human behavior in terms of continuous reciprocal interaction among cognitive, behavioral, and environmental influences.

Bobo doll viewing adults hitting the doll: Observational learning occurs through imitation **(Fig. 3.42)** of others. Bandura tested the children on imitation and observation by bobo doll experiment.

For example, the way we eat, drink, walk, talk, dress, etc., is all learnt by imitation. In learning process, major percentage depends on imitation. We observe and watch what and how other people do certain activities and imitate them.

The dance, music, yoga, etc., are learned by observation and imitation.

Episodic Learning

In episodic learning, incidents occur periodically and make people learn by this type of learning.

Transfer of learning: Transfer of learning is a process by which learning or training in one situation is carried over or transferred to other situation.

Crow and crow: New learning is based upon previously learned experience. People interpret new things in terms of what they already know. Transfer of learning refers to learning in one context and applying into another.

Types of Transfer of Learning

There are three types of transfer of learning **(Fig. 3.43)**:

1. **Positive transfer:** The classical dancer may feel easy to learn another type of dance by changing postures of body. The student who is good in mathematics feel easy to learn

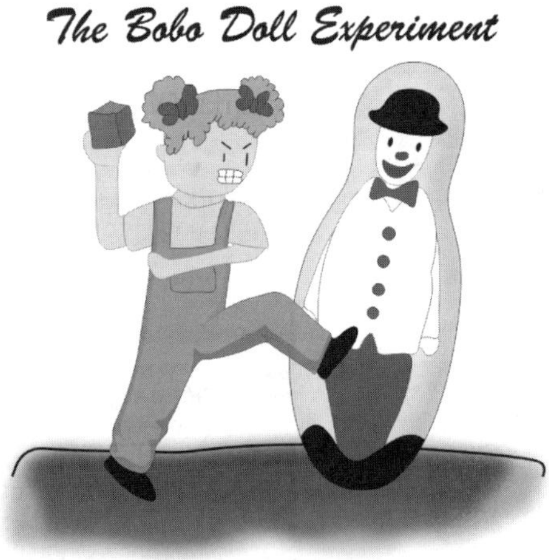

An experiment by Bandura (1961) in which adults modelled aggressive behavior towards a "Bobo doll"

• Children were observed to copy the adults.

• This supports Bandura's Social Learning Theory, which suggests people learn by observation, modelling, imitation, punishment and reward.

Fig. 3.42: Albert Bandura Social leaning process of Bobo doll

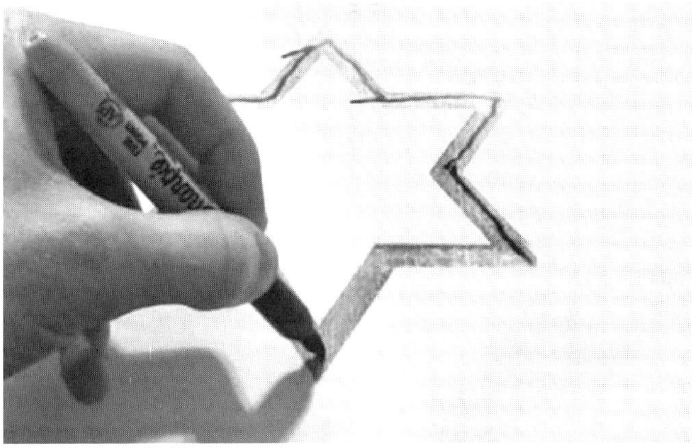

Fig. 3.43: Model of the transfer process

physics compared to the student who studied biological sciences. When learning in one situation facilitates learning in another situation, it is known as positive transfer.

2. **Negative transfer:** In negative transfer, the habit of learning in one process may feel difficult to change in short period of time. It is known as negative transfer. The child who learns to write English alphabets may feel difficult to manage writing Telugu letters. The changing of gears in motor vehicle and driving the wheels left side and right side may be difficult to manage, which are examples of negative transfer.
3. **Neutral transfer:** When learning of one activity neither facilitates nor hinders the learning of another task, it is a case of neutral transfer. It is also called as zero transfer. For example, knowledge of embroidery in no way affects learning of cooking in kitchen.

Study Habits

- Study skills—Study with definite purpose in mind.
- Manage to relax in meanwhile learning to reduce stress of continuity.
- Concentration is the essential point while learning.
- The effect of memory depends on rest and concentration.
- Sometimes note down the points while teaching or learning process.
- Apply and compare the matter into practical situations, if possible.
- Learning in a meaningful way may be easy to learn. Educators promote active recall, memorization and repetition. Rewrite the actual lecture notes or concept in one's own words.

MEMORY

Memory is very important process in day-to-day life. In psychology, an organism's ability to store and retain subsequently to retrieve information is known as memory.

Memory is a neurological process mediated by the brain that accounts for the capacity to retain and retrieve information. Memory is key cognitive ability to exercise judgment, make decisions, or even be oriented in time and place, a person remembers past experiences caused by good in memory process.

Definitions

James Drever: "Memory is the characteristic which underlines all learning, the essential feature of which is reflection. In narrow sense, it covers recall and recognition."

Maltin 2005: "Memory is the process of maintaining information over time."

Sternberg 1999: "Memory is the means by which we draw on our past experiences in order to use this information in the present."

Nature of Memory

- Learning and registration—Priority and guidance
- Retention—Preserved in brain
- Recall—Revival of past experience
- Recognition—Accepting the process

Learning or Registration

The cognitive process of memory depends on perfectness in learning and registering in mind based on priority and guidance. Our mind has a special ability by which every experience or learning leaves behind traces, which are conserved in the form of "engrains." This is known as learning.

Retention

The healthy functioning of nervous system is very important in retention. The engrains or memory traces are preserved in our brain with the help of our nervous system. This process is known as retention.

Recall

Recall means perfect revival of the past experiences. Recollection of information when we need is recall. It is difficult in recollecting some task or information due to lack of concentration while learning, stress, and mental illness. Recall is an active process.

Recognition

Recall and recognition are closely related. Recall provides material in memory, while recognition is the process of accepting or rejecting it. Recognition is more a passive behavior.

Development of Memory

In the development process of memory, there are three stages—encoding, storing, and retrieval **(Fig. 3.44)**.

Many experiments were designed to investigate memory but faced criticism due to less ecological validity. It is created in artificial manner to face reality. People are removed from their normal social settings and asked to take part in a psychological experiment.

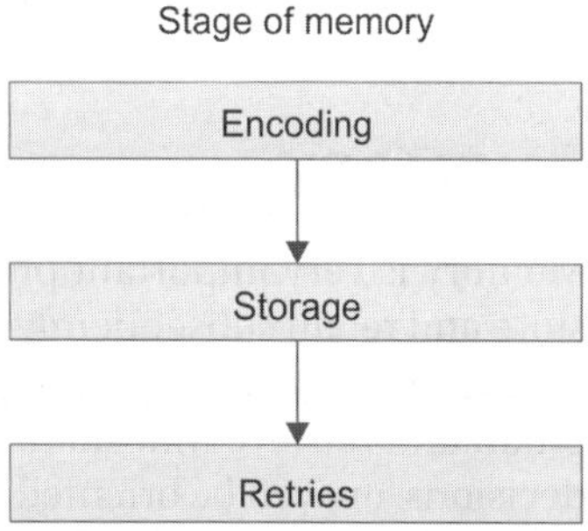

Fig. 3.44: Stages of memory

1. **Encoding:** Encoding is the process of getting information into the system by translating it into a neural code into

process of brain. The sensory information is stored in the form of different memory codes. Memory codes are the mental representation of physical stimuli. Encoding is receiving, processing, and combining all information. Encoding allows information from the outside world to be sensed in the form of chemical and physical stimuli. In the first stage, the information must be changed so that it may be put into the encoding process.

There are three main ways in which information can be encoded (changed):

- **Visual (picture):** Encoding that is represented as picture is called visual encoding, e.g. Remembering phone numbers from phone book, etc.
- **Acoustic (sound):** In this encoding, spoken words are represented in our mind in the form of sound. It is a short-term memory. The individual can hold in memory by rehearsing verbally.
- **Semantic (meaning):** The information in LTM can also be coded both visually and acoustically.

2. **Storing:** Storage is the second memory stage or process. In this process, information is maintained over short periods of time. In this process, memory store STM or LTM depends on capacity, quality, and duration, and time of information is important. The way we store information affects retrieval.

   Most adults can store between 5 and 9 items in their short-term memory. Miller (1956) put this idea forward and he called it the magic number 7. He thought that short-term memory capacity was 7 (plus or minus 2) items because it only had a certain number of "slots" in which items could be stored.

   However, Miller did not specify the amount of information that can be held in each slot. Indeed, if we can "chunk" information together, we can store a lot more information in our short-term memory. In contrast, the capacity of LTM is thought to be unlimited.

   Information can only be stored for a brief duration in STM (0–30 seconds), but LTM can last a life time.

3. **Retrieval:** Some retrieval attempts may be effortless due to the type of information, and other attempts to remember stored information may be more demanding for various reasons.

   Some of the information may not recall back due to various reasons. STM is stored and retrieved sequentially. For example, if a group of participants is given a list of words to remember, and then asked to recall the fourth word on the list, participants go through the list in the order they heard it in previously to retrieve the information.

LTM is stored and retrieved by association. Organizing information can help aid retrieval. The sequences in storing information can be organized by size, time, and alphabetical order, for example, discharged patient following the instructions of doctor in taking medicines, suggestions to speedy recovery like dressing, exercise etc. Forgetting can be possible by brain damage.

Types of Memory (Fig. 3.45)

1. Immediate memory or sensory memory
2. Short-term memory (STM)
3. Long-term memory (LTM).

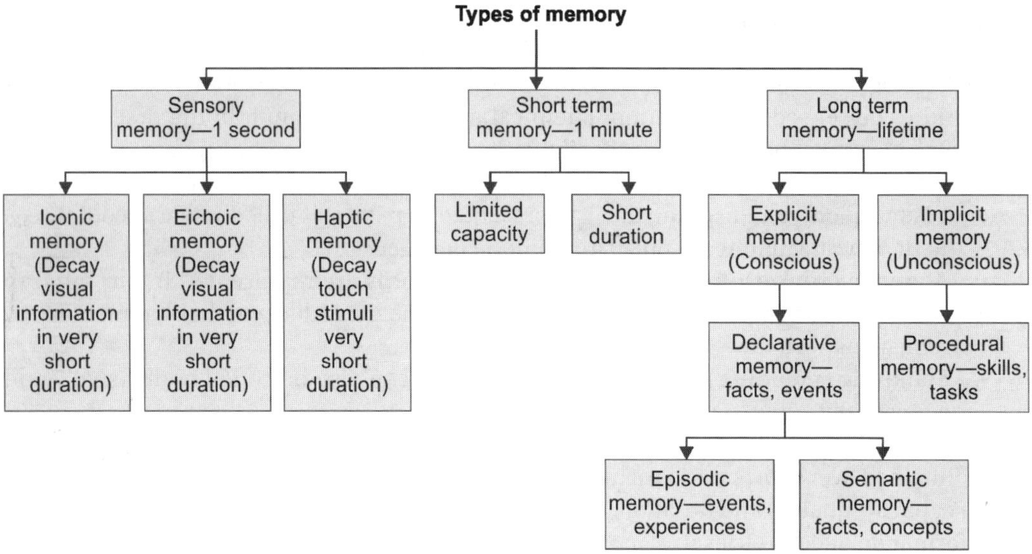

Fig. 3.45: Types of human memory

Sensory Memory

The term sensory refers to initial process of storing information that is perceived through our **senses**. It lasts for some period of time and is regularly replaced by new data continuously. Sensory memory is memorised for a split second without cognitive control and responding automatically. This type of memory cannot be prolonged via rehearsal.

Three types of sensory memory

i. **Iconic memory:** Iconic memory is decaying visual information very fast. In this type of Iconic memory is decaying visual information very fast.
ii. **Echoic memory:** Echoic memory is a fast decaying store of auditory information. It perceives sounds or auditory information for a short period.
iii. **Haptic memory:** Haptic memory is a type of sensory memory that represents a database for touch stimuli.

Short-term Memory

Short-term memory is known as working memory. It allows to recall for limited duration supported by transient patterns of neuronal communication, dependent on regions of frontal lobe and the parietal lobe.

It is decayed very early by lack of rehearsal. The individual may feel difficult to recall more information in a limited period. The person's memory is strong by repetition or exercise in proceeding of long-term memory.

The short-term memory is improved by adaptation of chunking and rehearsal process.

- **Chunking:** Chunking enables us to recall information in groups which greatly increase the capacity of short-term memory. It is possible to recall by dividing into parts or groups rather than a major group or more pieces of information. For example, remembering telephone number by trying to divide it into two or three, to recall it fast, is called chunking. This is because we can chunk the information into meaningful groups of numbers.

This may be reflected in some countries in the tendency to display telephone numbers as several chunks of two to four numbers.

- **Rehearsal:** In this process, we repetitively verbalize or think about the information. This short-term memory duration is also limited. The decay of stored information is due to lack of rehearsal. It disappears fast and feels difficult to remember the information due to lack of rehearsal.

Long-term Memory

The storage in sensory memory and short-term memory generally has a strictly limited capacity and duration, which means that information is not retained indefinitely.

The difference between long-term memory and short-term memory: In long-term memory, stored information will remain strong in memory for a long duration (sometimes for whole life span). While short-term memory encodes information acoustically, long-term memory encodes it semantically: Another part of long-term memory is episodic memory, which attempts to capture information such as "what," "when," and where, with episodic memory, individuals are able to recall specific events such as birthday parties and weddings. Long-term memory, on the other hand, is maintained by more stable and permanent changes in neural connections widely spread throughout the brain.

Explicit Memory or Declarative Memory

Declarative memory involves both episodic and semantic memory. Episodic memory and semantic memory are two major types of memories that make up part of your long-term memory; together they are known as declarative memory.

Episodic Memory

In this type of memory, people can recall details of event and experience in discriminative way for a long period. It is possible for analyzation of every event or experience without difficulty. But some information may have decayed without being registered into long period. The researchers believe that emotions play a major role in this process of memory.

Episodic memory is a person's unique memory of a specific event, so it will be different from someone else's recollection of the same experience.

Episodic memory is sometimes confused with autobiographical memory. It also relies on semantic memory. For example, the name of the city, birthday dates, and details of family relations are automatically specific in our memory.

Examples of episodic memory

- The first time flight journey
- First day in college
- First day of new job
- First day meeting of life partner
- First meeting with a celebrity.

Semantic Memory

Semantic memory includes things that are common in recall such as names of states, their capitals, identification of quality of sounds, remembering letters, symbols, etc. Semantic memory is just the facts.

Some examples of semantic memory include:

- The color of crow is black.
- Recall the list of National holidays and specific dates, etc., e.g. August 15th Independence day.
- Traffic signals, red is danger to cross the road, Green is safe, etc.

Implicit Memory or Procedural Memory

These memories are unconscious in recall. The past experience is cause for recalling in short duration. Procedural memory is primarily employed in learning motor skills and should be considered a subset of implicit. For example, in the learning of driving, usage of things in proper direction is considered as implicit memory.

Procedural memory involved in motor learning depends on the cerebrum and ganglia.

Musicians and professional athletes are said to have superior ability to form procedural memories. Some examples of procedural memory include the ability to ride a bike, play guitar, piano, etc. It is possible by rehearsal several times and past experience. Procedural memory is a subset of implicit memory and is a part of the long-term memory, for example, the operation of instruments and driving are motor skills. The circumstances make to respond without rehearsal in implicit memory.

Examples of procedural memory

- Playing musical instruments
- Usage of bats and balls in games and sports
- Swimming
- Skating
- Climbing trees, etc.
- Implicit memory depends on explicit memory in efforts of tracing the surface of correct path.

Factors Influencing Memory Process

Memory is stated as a process which includes learning, retention, and remembering. The change is noticed in physical activities and behavioral process (**Fig. 3.46**).

Intrinsic factorss
Age
Interest
Intelligence
Medical conditions (blood pressure, brain tumors, Alzheimers, addiction of alohol, drugs

Factors influencing memory

Extrinsic factor
Quantity of matierial
Verbal or non–verbal
Distractions
Physical conditions

Fig. 3.46: Factors influencing memory

Intrinsic Factors

Age, interest, intelligence, medical conditions (blood pressure, brain tumors, Alzheimer's, addiction to alcohol, drugs, etc.).

Age is one of the criteria in memory. In most of the research, the memory raises sharp in age between 16 and 26 compared to elders.

Interest on specific areas is strong in memory by their learning process. Frequency of applying gives no chance of decaying.

Intelligence is very important in grasping theme, necessity for long duration in memory.

- **Medical condition:** Medical factors such as usage of medicines without guidance of medical professional, wrong usage of drugs, and insufficiency of intakes with medicines may influence on physical and psychological functioning of body and mind. Sometimes, it may have causes that negatively affect memory change: medical disorders and diseases (thyroid problems, heart problems, stroke).
- **Emotional problems:** Emotional fluctuations may cause improper conditions of memory. Negative emotions like distress, depression, over anxiety, medication (some anti-depressants) and stimulants may have influence on body and mind for loss of memory.

Extrinsic Factor

Quantity of material, verbal or non-verbal, and distractions.

The material and quality impress human mind to create interest in store and remember the whole in a short duration by its color, size, and contrast dominate other in grasping and the purpose for a long duration in memory. The meaningful material draws human attention in arousing interest in learning, retaining, and reproducing the material.

Verbal or non-verbal communication influences our memory by good voice, or speech by their pronunciation; clarity on theme attracts our attention toward strong in memory.

Non-verbal communication creates interest in memory by photography, script, scenery, painted colors in contrast, dazzling lighting, and publicity which may register fast and strong in storage.

Distraction creates lack of interest in memory. It is very difficult to grasp due to irritation or louder noise, unsuitable atmosphere, and other problems linked to lapse of memory.

Good physical health: The changes in body functioning and hormonal changes in adolescence, for example, menopause in ladies, cause a change in memory levels (high and low). Elderly people may suffer Alzheimer's disease. Poor diet (high fat, too high cholesterol, too low cholesterol) may cause of loss in memory. Loss of memory is known as amnesia. Amnesia can result from extensive damage to the regions of the medial temporal lobe.

Physical exercise, particularly continuous aerobic exercises such as running, cycling, and swimming, has many cognitive benefits and effects on the brain. The effects of exercise on memory have important implications for improving children's academic performance, maintaining mental abilities in old age, and the prevention and potential cure of neurological diseases.

Social factors: Competition in society helps to improve memory by comparing with others in school, business, employment, and farming; in practice, hard work may influence on memory and recall the process to implement in day-to-day life.

Other factors: Sleep and rest and good diet are main factors for good memory.

Best Methods to Improve Memory

- **Repeated recitation:** Repetition is very important technique to improve memory. Repeating the difficult word several times will will become easy to pronounce. Most of the shlokas in Sanskrit will become easy to pronounce fluently by daily practice. The non-sense syllables are replaced by sensible material; we get better results. Recitation is a greater advantage for permanent memory than for immediate memory.
- **Whole versus part learning:** Memorizing major paragraphs or large scale of work by division of parts is called whole versus part learning. In this process of memory, prepare some simple tips in separation using a symbol, alphabets, digits, or numbers to recall for details of information into full fledge. The "part method" yields good results from immediate memory.
- **The spaced learning:** This type of learning depends on giving gap in each trial of learning. The rest is also an important tip in rehearsals for a long duration. Spaced learning yields better result for permanent memory. Unspaced learning is good for immediate memory.

Meaningful Learning Memory

The meaning and understanding of theme and the connectivity of the order of task is easy to keep in mind, and it leads to effective memorization. On the other hand, intelligent memorizing of a sensible material in which the connected meaning of the whole matter is grasped is far more effective.

Intention of Memory

Learning a matter effectively requires the intention to remember. The will to learn is necessary if any learning is to be accomplished. They can remember those things only which they noted and intended to remember. Unintentional learning is ineffective cause for loss of memory. We can learn a list of 50 non-sense syllables by reading it some hundreds of times. But even in learning a list of non-sense syllables, we should have the intention to learn it.

The Method of Loci

The word loci mean "places." The memory that depends on the system of recalling the address of street, or building visualized by description in mind to trace out is a loci method of learning.

- **Mnemonics:** Mnemonics comes from the Greek word for memory and refers to the specific memory improvement techniques. Most mnemonics techniques rely on the linking or association of to be remembered material with a systematic and organized set of images or words with which we are familiar, and therefore can provide reminder cues.
- **Chunking:** Chunking is remembering the important dates and phone numbers associated with significant number by breaking into chunks, i.e. remembering pin numbers of debit cards, etc.

Simple Tips of Memory in Studying

- Study schedule
- Rehearsal
- Priority
- New ways of thinking

- Reduction of stress
- Nutritious food
- Good sleep
- Exercise
- Restriction of drugs, smoking, alcohol, etc.

Did you know??

A UCLA (University of California in Los Angeles) research study published in the June 2006.

A UCLA (University of California in Los Angeles) research study published in the June 2006 issue of the *American Journal of Geriatric Psychiatry* found that people can improve cognitive function and improve brain efficiency through simple lifestyle changes such as incorporating memory exercises, healthy eating, physical fitness, and stress reduction into their daily lives. This study examined 17 subjects (average age 53) with normal memory performance. Eight subjects were asked to follow a "brain healthy" diet, relaxation, physical, and mental exercise (brain teasers and verbal memory training techniques). After 14 days, they showed greater word fluency (not memory) compared to their baseline performance. No long-term follow-up was conducted; it is therefore unclear if this intervention has lasting effects on memory.

Forgetting

The loss of memory is described as forgetfulness or amnesia. Forgetting is common in part of daily life.

Forgetting is generally not losing or erasing the information from our long-term memory. The individual may feel difficult to recall information which is called forgetting. It is common in all ages of people. Some people may recall in brief duration, but other people recall it back for a long duration. It depends on several factors of age, medical conditions, psychological problems, and malfunctioning of brain. Forgetting typically involves failure in memory retrieval. While the information is somewhere in our long-term memory, we are not able to retrieve and remember it.

Munn 1967: "Forgetting is defined as the permanent or temporary loss of the ability to recall or recognize something learned earlier."

Bhatia: "Forgetting is the failure of the individual to revive in consciousness an idea or group of ideas without the help of the original stimulus."

Psychologist Hermann Ebbinghaus was one of the first to be scientifically studied about forgetting. In experiments where he used himself as the subject, Ebbinghaus tested his memory using three-letter non-sense syllables. They did not use these previously. He came to conclusion that previously used words would have involved drawing on his existing knowledge and associations in his memory.

In order to test for new information, Ebbinghaus tested his memory for periods of time ranging from 20 minutes to 31 days. He then published his findings in 1885.

Memory: "A contribution to experimental psychology."

Strategies for Forgetfulness

- **Recall:** People who have been asked to memorize something, such as a list of terms, might be asked to recall the list from memory. The quantity, number of items to recall, and meaningful ways are also important points in proving efforts in forgetfulness.

- **Recognition:** This method involves identifying information that was previously learned. On a test, for example, students might have to recognize which terms they learned about in a chapter of their assigned reading.

Causes of Forgetting

1. Retrieval failure
2. Interference
3. Failure to store
4. Motivated forgetting.

Theories of Forgetting

The Interference Theory of Forgetting

According to interference theory, forgetting is the result of different memories interfering with one another. The changing methods of frequency by following new also cause forgetting. It is very difficult to recall due to replacement of the new method which gives chance to forget the previous very easily.

Interference: It was assumed that memory can be disrupted or interfered with new ideas which suggests that information in long-term memory may become confused or combined with other information during encoding, thus distorting or disrupting memories.

Unique and distinctive events like merit in studies, wedding, and birth dates are much more likely to be recalled in a very easy way. Serial of priority is also another cause of forgetfulness. In most of the cases, the first and last items or tasks are good in process of memory.

Proactive interference: The previously learned information makes it more difficult to form new memories. Learning a new phone number or locker combination might be more difficult, for example, because our memories of our old phone number and combination interfere with the new information.

Retroactive interference occurs when we forget a previously learnt task due to the leaning of new task. In other words, later learning interferes with earlier learning—where new memories disrupt old memories.

Proactive and retroactive interference is thought to be more likely to occur where the memories are similar, for example: confusing old and new telephone numbers. Chandler (1989) stated that students who study similar subjects at the same time often experience interference.

The Trace Decay Theory of Forgetting

According to the trace theory of memory, the formation of new memories results in physical and chemical changes in the brain that result in a memory "trace." This theory suggests that short-term memory can only hold information for 15 to 30 seconds unless it is rehearsed. After this time, the information/trace decays and fades away. Trace theory states that forgetting occurs as a result of the automatic decay or fading of the memory trace. Trace decay theory focuses on tie and the limited duration of short-term memory.

According to the trace decay theory of forgetting, the events that happen between the formation of a memory and the recall of the memory have no impact on recall. Instead, trace theory proposes that is the length of time between the memory and recalling that information determines whether the information will be retained or forgotten. If the time interval is short, more information will be recalled. If a longer period passes, more information will be forgotten and memory will be poorer.

The idea that memories fade over time is hardly new. The Greek philosopher Plato suggested such a thing more than 2,500 years ago. Later, experimental research by psychologists such as Ebbinghaus bolstered this theory.

Another problem with decay theory is effect of faded memories very fast while some memories are longer. Novelty is one factor that plays a role in remembering and forgetting.

The Retrieval Failure Theory

Retrieval failure is where the information is in long-term memory, but cannot be accessed. Such information is said to be available (i.e. it is still stored) but not accessible (i.e. it cannot be retrieved). It cannot be accessed because the retrieval cues are not present.

When we store a new memory, we are also storing information about the situation and these are known as retrieval cues. When we come into the same situation again, these retrieval cues can trigger the memory of the situation.

Sometimes the individual may feel difficult to access in mind. Two of the basic reasons for this failure in memory retrieval are related to encoding failures and lack of retrieval cues.

The Cue-Dependent Theory of Forgetting

Some of the researchers have found that the information which is present in memory cannot be recalled unless retrieval cues are present. These cues are elements that were present at the time that the actual memory was encoded. For example, remembering the details of our first day in the college with our classmate might be easier than the other events on that day.

Amnesia

Amnesia is referring to an inability to recall information that is stored in memory. In simple terms, amnesia is the loss of memory. The cause of amnesia is based on organic or functional process of memory of an individual. Organic cause of amnesia may include brain damage through injury, or the use of specific drugs or sedatives.

Amnesia is one of the symptoms of some degenerative brain diseases, such as Alzheimer's disease. Functional cause of amnesia **(Fig. 3.47)** is based on psychological factors, genetic defects, etc. The defense mechanisms may be applied in some of the frustrated situation to get temporary relief from distress.

Types of Amnesia (Fig. 3.48)

Biological Amnesia

Anterograde amnesia: The patient cannot remember new information compared to the storage of strong long memory. It depends on age and some other reasons, for example, to accept new ideas and to adjust in modern circumstances. Things that happened recently should be stored into short-term memory and disappear very quickly by lack of application. This is usually caused by brain trauma (brain damage from a blow to the head, for example). A patient with anterograde amnesia can remember data and events which happened before the injury.

Retrograde amnesia: Often thought of as the opposite of anterograde amnesia. The patient cannot remember events that occurred before his/her trauma, but he or she remembers things that happened after it normally.

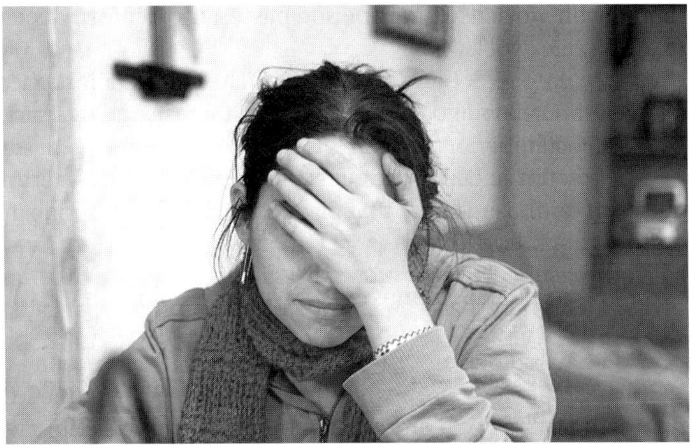

Fig. 3.47: Suffering with amnesia

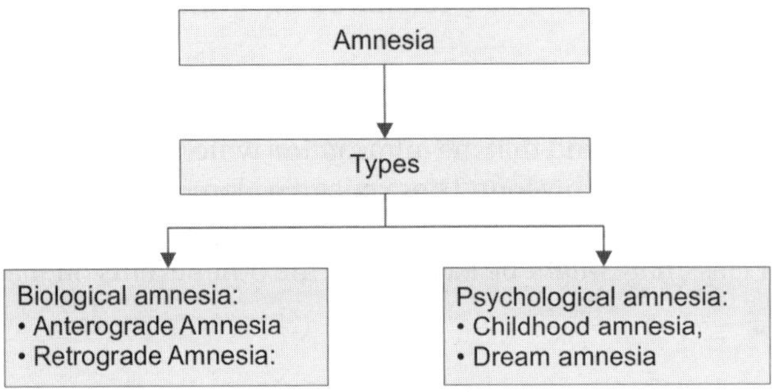

Fig. 3.48: Types of amnesia

Psychological Amnesia

- **Childhood amnesia (infantile amnesia):** The patient cannot recall events from early childhood. Experts say this type of amnesia may be associated with language development. Others say it is possible that some memory areas of the brain were not fully mature during childhood.
- **Dream amnesia:** In dream amnesia, the difference between the symbol system in dreams and in waking makes the waking retrieval of any information encoded during dream difficult.
- **Dementia:** Dementia refers to a large class of disorders characterized by the progressive deterioration of thinking ability and memory as the brain becomes damaged. Dementia can be categorized as reversible (thyroid disease) or irreversible (Alzheimer disease).

Methods to Improve Memory

- Paper learning method
- Method of loci
- Rhyming system
- Make a story
- Chunking
- Overlearning.

Simple Tips for Good Memory

- Study to work
- Rehearsal
- Feedback
- Review.

THINKING

Thinking is essential in all forms of cognitive processes like perception, learning, memory, and aptitude. Sometimes the term thinking is an important in solution of problems, creating with new ideas.

Our brains have evolved to meet certain important demands, and many of their functions may be subserved by especially evolved, relatively autonomous systems. The mind helps in creating new ideas, thinking, processing information, forming concepts, and problem solving by analyzing the reasons in decision-making.

Thinking is an organized, systematic, goal-oriented activity. Thinking is an activity in humans by strengthening their relationship between stimulus and response. It can be interpreted in recalling information and its consequences.

Thinking is a conscious process and activates mind to make new connections in creative ideas toward the purpose of topic. It has the quality of an internal conversation between different perspectives.

Thinking is a process of gathering information and helps in psychological and physical well-being of the individuals. It also helps cognitively by rearranging the information from the environment and symbols are stored in the memory of its past. Cognitive abilities like thinking, reasoning, and problem-solving may be considered to be some of the chief characteristics which distinguish human beings from other species including the higher animals **(Fig. 3.49)**. The powers of thinking and reasoning may be considered to be the essential tools for the welfare and meaningful existence of the individual as well as society.

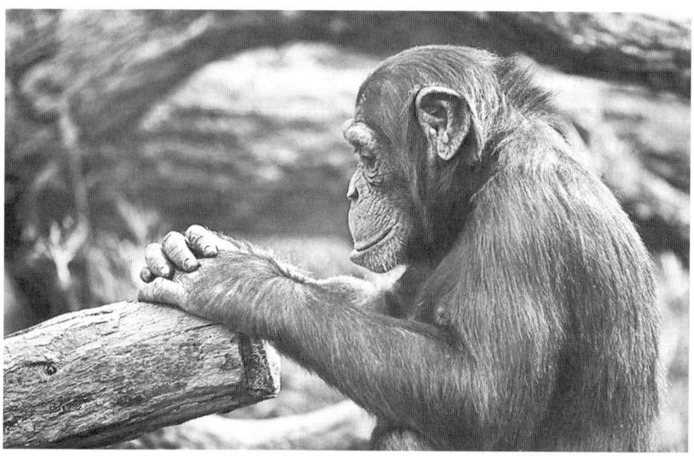

Fig. 3.49: A chimpanzee thinking

Definition

Whittaker: Whittaker defines that "thinking is a complex cognitive form of behavior which occurs only at relatively advanced stage of development when simpler and more direct methods of dealing with the environment have proved ineffective".

Ross (1951): Thinking is mental activity in its cognitive aspect or mental activity with regard to psychological objects.

Maier: Thinking is a higher mental process involving symbols, images, concepts, and ideas that mediate between stimuli and response.

Gilmer (1970): "Thinking is a problem solving process in which we use ideas or symbols in place of overt activity."

Types of Thinking

- Perceptual or concrete thinking
- Conceptual or abstract thinking
- Creative thinking
- Reasoning or logical thinking
- Problem solving.

Perceptual or Concrete Thinking

This is the simplest form of thinking based on perception. It is like presentation of sensation according to one's experience. It is an interpretation of sensation expressed by an experience of human life. It is also called concrete thinking and carried out over perception of actual objects and events. It is benefited mainly for young children.

Conceptual or Abstract Thinking

This type of thinking does not require actual objects or events. It needs concepts. It is superior to perceptual thinking and economizes efforts in understanding, helping in discovery and investigation. It is based on generalized ideas and languages. Language plays an important role in conceptual thinking.

Creative Thinking

Creative thinking is based on novelty or newness. It is a type of research or invention for new solutions. It provides new relationship to describe or interpret the nature of things or circumstances in getting solutions for problems. So it is called creative thinking.
Example: Scientists, artists, and inventors.

Characteristics of Creative Thinking

- Creative thinking gives some mental task toward newness. It is very important in cognitive behavior.
- Every individual is capable of thinking and making it into process of interpretation. It forms to fulfilment of activities.
- Creative thinking also results in production and investments in a variety of forms including a new form of arrangement of old elements.
- It builds new personality by motivating the individual in creation. It covers all the aspects of human necessities belonging to an individual's life.

- Creative thinking in all its dimensions involves divergent thinking instead of the routine and final types of convergent thinking. Creative thinking is defined as personal, imaginative thinking which produces a new, novel, and useful solution. Creative thinking is divergent thought and not convergent thought.

Divergent thinking: This type of thinking begins from a common goal and moves out into a variety of perspectives.

Convergent thinking: This type of thinking is cognitive process of information around a common goal. It is an attempt for new thoughts converting into different directions with common conclusion.

The processes involved in creative thinking are studied through the reports of great thinkers and inventors. Interviews, questionnaires, and introspective reports are based on common purpose. Creative thinking involves the following steps **(Fig. 3.50)**:

- Preparation
- Incubation
- Illumination
- Evaluation
- Revision.
- **Preparation:** Preparation involves formulation of the problem and collection of necessary and relevant data in getting solutions.
- **Incubation** occurs when the individual may have experience that provides clues to the solutions.
- **Illumination:** Illumination is the final stage in creative problem solving. In this process, sudden thoughts click in mind while problem solving.
- **Evaluation:** Illumination is followed by evaluation. It is a verification for full process of data collected and kept into form. It is also useful for slight modification.
- **Revision:** It is the final step in the process of creative thinking. It is perfect after all processing stages.

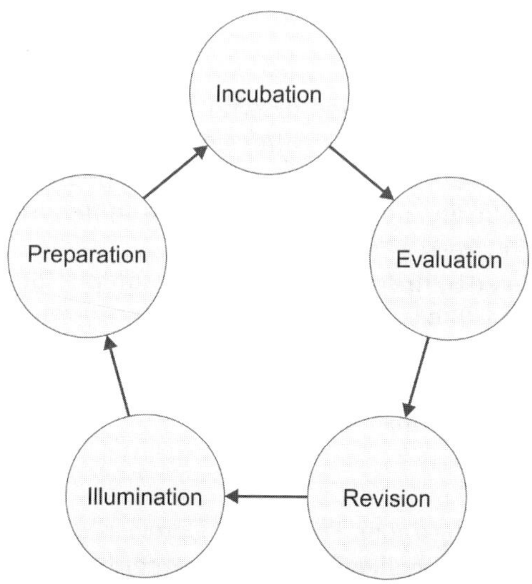

Fig. 3.50: Steps in creative thinking

Free Thinking

This is also called as free-floating thinking. This is more common among children. There is no chance for reality in this form of thinking. Generally, such thinking will be highly private and the individual may use symbols with very personal meanings.

Types of free thinking

- **Fantasy:** It is called as daydreaming, dreaming in an awaken state. In this type, people imagine different scenes in their mind and feel pleasure. There is no limitation in daydreaming. It is also one type of defense mechanism. Examples: People imagine them as their favorite hero or heroine, a merit student may imagine him as gold medalist, and a player may imagine him as getting shield in his career. Even the impossible things become possible by fantasy or daydreaming. But too much of daydreaming may make him incapable of facing reality.
- **Dreaming:** Sigmund Freud has stated that the dreams are wish fulfillments. Our desires which are not fulfilled in real appear in the form of dreams and to fulfill. There are no restrictions or limitations for appearance of these dreams. They may appear directly or in disguise form.
- **Imagination:** Imagination is a mental activity like dreaming. In the process of imagination, there is no sense of perception. These are only mental images.

Controlled Thinking

The controlled thinking is a creativity for newness to get solutions. Our thoughts will be in touch with reality and clarity in the thinking based on goal.

Forms of Controlled Thinking

Reasoning:

Reasoning is one of the best forms of controlled thinking. It is direct conscious process of thinking toward problem solutions. It depends on factual data.

Mann (1967): "Reasoning is combining past experience to solve a problem, which cannot be solved by mere reproduction of earlier solutions."

Reasoning is of two types:

1. **Inductive reasoning:** Inductive logic (reasoning) arrives at general principle based on particular instances. So, the conclusion drawn is wider than premises, e.g., we arrive at a conclusion that all politicians are selfish after seeing many politicians.
2. **Deductive reasoning:** Deductive logic (reasoning) depends on valid conclusions from assumptions, e.g., socratic and derived solutions. It is shifted from universal to individual. All men are mortal. All actresses are beautiful.

Thinking is also influenced by the mode of reason one adopts. Illogical reasoning often leads to incorrect thinking. Logic is the science of correct reasoning which helps to think correctly. Therefore, we should cultivate the habit of logical reasoning among our children.

Generally, in reasoning, logical principles are applied to our thinking. It will be most directed toward getting at certain conclusions and inferences.

Problem Solving

A problem is a barrier in reaching a goal. The thinking process starts in problem solving to reach a goal. A goal can be reached by recollecting previous experiences in problem solving. Problem solving can be done by trial and error or by insight.

John Deway has suggested a scientific method of problem solving which follows the following procedure

- Recognizing the problem
- Defining the problem
- Collection of relevant data
- Formulation of hypothesis
- Evaluation of hypothesis
- Verification
- Conclusions.

Stages of Thinking or Levels of Thinking

- **Analyzation:** Analyzation involves thinking about a whole in terms of its various parts. We can encourage this level of thinking by asking children what materials could be used for a classroom project.
- **Comparison and confirmation** involve looking at the meaning of the knowledge that has been gathered and drawing conclusions from it.
- **Applying:** Entails using what has been learned in new situations. Asking children to consider a newly learned fact as they build or make something can do faster in this level of thinking.
- **Evaluating** entails making comparisons and judgments. We can encourage this level of thinking by asking children which of the materials they used for being best in performance.

Development of Thinking

Thinking is one of the most important aspects of learning process. Our ability to learn and solve the problems depends upon our ability to think correctly which helps us in adjustment and necessary for a successful living.

The development of every process depends on planning procedure, experience, and interpretation. The motivation starts by interest and necessity of the particular process and benefits of achievement.

Flexibility

The success may be difficult in some of the circumstances not cooperated in reaching goal. The thinking process may be diverted to choose another way to get success. The restrictions are also barriers in development. Proper care should be taken to use intelligence, wisdom, and other cognitive abilities for carrying out the process of thinking.

Tools of Thinking

There are a few important elements involved in the thinking process:

- **Images:** Images are objects, situations what they experience in day-to-day life. The mental pictures are used in thinking, manipulating rather than the actual objects, experiences, or activities.
- **Concepts:** A concept is a general idea that stands for a general class and represents the common characteristics of all objects or events of this general class.
- **Symbols and signs:** Symbols and signs represent and stand for substitute of the actual objects, experiences, and activities. For example, traffic lights and different sounds of vehicle

horns like ambulance, fire engines, etc. Badges of national flag and different political parties represent their aims.

- **Language:** Language is the most efficient and developed vehicle used for carrying out the process of thinking. When a person reads, writes, or hears words or sentences or observes gesture in any language, one is stimulated to think. Thus, reading and writing of documents and literature also help in stimulating and promoting the thinking process.

Relationship between Language and Communication

The interrelationship of thought and language is an extremely complex problem. The concept thought content is integral to the expressive theory of linguistic communication. Contents conceived as something shared in communication must be distinguished from contents of various other kinds represented in philosophical literature.

Tools of Communication

- Language
- Observation and perception
- Nonverbal behavior
- Silence
- Listening
- Watching.

Development of Concepts and Language

Concept is a word or idea with a generalized meaning which represents an entire class of objects, ideas, or events. Concept is an important situation in which subject learns to make an identifying response to members which are not completely identical stimuli.

Language is the chief vehicle of communication. It depends on images, symbols, muscle, and brain activities which are more essential in developmental process.

Language is classified into two forms, verbal and nonverbal communications.

Verbal language is a means of communication. Verbal communication involves the spoken or written word. Verbal language is a code that conveys specific meaning as words are combined. It depends on vocabulary, clarity of voice, etc.

In psychology, language and communication are more valuable in assessing personality and intelligence. Psychologists are now agreeing that language could form part or even majority of our declarative memory, or that component of our long-term memory that comprises ideas and information that can be verbally communicated.

Muscular Activities

Thinking in one way or the other shows the evidence of the involvement of some incipient movements of groups of our muscles. All individuals are different in postures of walking, running, standing, and sitting. These may change muscular tensions and contraversions. People can control these muscle activities by exercise, yoga or meditation, and different dances.

Brain Functions

Whatever may be the role of the muscles, thinking is primarily a function of the brain. Our mind is said to be the chief instrument of the thinking process. The experiences registered by our sense organs have no meaning, and thus cannot serve as stimulating agents or instruments for thinking unless these impressions are received by our brain cells and properly interpreted to derive some meaning.

The mental pictures or images can be stored, reconstructed, or used only on being processed by the brain.

Errors in Thinking

Errors in thinking depend on our thinking, reasoning, and problem-solving behavior which all are largely influenced by our "sets." It is also common in individual attitudes, likes, and dislikes. These mental sets that have been gained from previous experiences surely interfere with our subsequent thinking resulting in ineffective behavior. Sometimes we make false statements and develop prejudice and conflicts without noticing the facts. The errors in thinking may also cause to distorted by superstitions or by lack of information that is relevant to the subject.

INTELLIGENCE

Human intelligence is a mental activity consisting of abilities or skills learned by experience. It helps to manage new situations by learned knowledge toward problem solutions. The word intelligence is derived from the Latin verb "Intellegere" means understanding. Intelligence involves some different mental abilities including logic, reasoning, problem-solving, and planning.

In a 1921 symposium, the American psychologists, Lewis M Termon and Edward L Thorndike differed over the definition of intelligence.

Definitions

Alfred Binet: "Intelligence is the ability for judgment or common sense."

Thorndike: "Intelligence is one's capacity to deal effectively with situations."

Jean Piaget: "Intelligence is the ability to adapt to one's surroundings."

Cyril Burt: "Intelligence is the capacity of flexible adjustment."

David Wechsler (1977): "The global capacity to think rationally, act purposefully, and deal effectively with the environment."

Intelligence is defined as mental capability that involves the ability to reason, to plan, to solve problems, to think abstractly, to comprehend complex ideas, to learn quickly, and to learn from experience. It is not merely book learning, a narrow academic skill, or test-taking smartness. Intelligence is an individual personality characteristic.

Classification of Intelligence

Intelligence is classified into three categories **(Fig. 3.51)**.

1. **Abstract intelligence:** It is developed by studying of books in different subjects and referred in large scale of their study. The scholars, eminent lawyers, and doctors are having abstract intelligence. A person with abstract intelligence is able to discover relations among symbols to solve problems, i.e. professionals like doctors, lawyers, and literacy men.
2. **Social intelligence:** Social intelligence of individual is developed by social interactions. The social interaction is agencies of parents, neighborhood, school, religion, and state. The

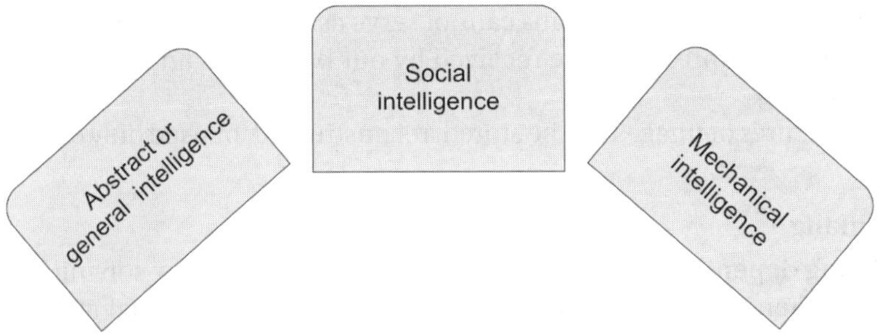

Fig. 3.51: Classification of intelligence

individual personality is also developed by using of intelligence according to necessities of the individual. The modification behavior of individual is also possible by adjustment even in the complicated situations by choosing intelligent ideas. Most of the politicians are getting success by technique of social intelligence to please the public to get success in winning votes from public. Therefore, intelligence is an inborn ability of an individual, and the distribution of intelligence is not equal among all human beings. There is wide individual difference that exists among individuals about intelligence. The developmental period of intelligence is from birth to adolescence.

There is a minor difference in the development of intelligence between boys and girls. There are individual differences about the intelligence between boys and girls.

The intelligence is determined by heredity and also shined through suitable environment.

3. **Mechanical intelligence:** This intelligence is individual's ability of knowledge in connection to the facts in day-to-day life. Most of the professionals like engineers and architects use their skills for novelty in their working areas. There is choice of choosing new techniques which are more profitable and valuable in their profession. They will use concrete objects to get success.

Artificial Intelligence

Artificial intelligence (AI) is a branch of computer science related to machine intelligence that studies to mimic (imitate person) to the "cognitive" function of human brain and mind. AI demonstrates to design software and hardware equipment that has abilities of learning, reasoning, analyzing, problem-solving capabilities, speech recognition, computer vision, etc., without supervision or extremely little supervision.

AI has spanned to a most intelligible science that could be used by mankind and already being used in precision healthcare (used by medical experts), banking and forex, business, and social networking.

Unlike AI, machine learning is a capability of AI given to a machine or software that is equal to capacity and intelligence of at least 100 human brains not just one human brain stimulation.

Theories of Intelligence

Charles Spearman—General Intelligence

British psychologist Charles Spearman (1863–1945) described the concept of general intelligence. Fundamentals on intellectual functioning are the influence of "G" or general factor and the presence of various special abilities as "S" is responsible for the relationships and their existence **(Fig. 3.52)**. They are musical or athletic skills. Spearman concluded that

Early theories of Intelligence

- Charles Spearman
  - Believed intelligence is general –"g-factor"
  - People who are bright in one area are usually bright in other areas as well
- L.L. Thurstone
  - Believed that intelligence is made up of seven distinct, independent abilities: spatial ability, perceptual speed, numerical ability, verbal meaning, memory, word fluency, reasoning
  - Did not believe in a g-factor, but those who scored well in one of the seven areas tended to score well on others.

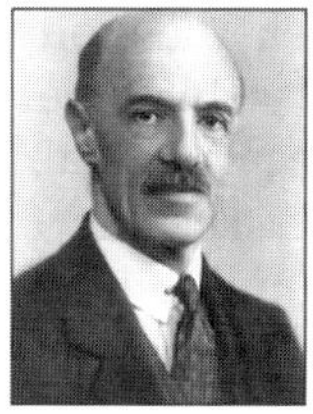

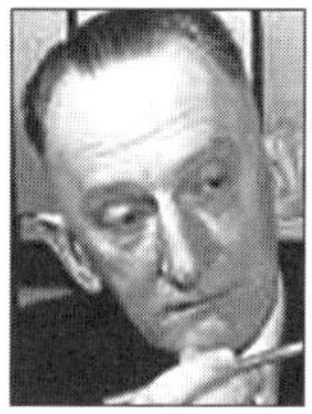

Fig. 3.52: Early theorist of Intelligence Spearman and Thurstone

every score on these tests was remarkable in general, which is universal, and a specific S is a factor that is found in each test alone. For example, an arithmetic test might tap both G and S, a specific mathematical ability. The measuring score of the IQ is closely related to the Spearman's idea of intelligence consisting of one general ability factor. These are included in visual-spatial processing, quantitative reasoning, knowledge, fluid reasoning, and working memory.

Louis L Thurstone—Primary Mental Abilities

Psychologist Louis L Thurstone (1887–1955) offered a theory of intelligence. Instead of viewing intelligence as a single, general ability, Thurstone's theory focused on seven different "primary mental abilities."

Primary mental abilities described by Thurstone (Fig. 3.52)

- Verbal comprehension—Ability to grasp meaning of words
- Reasoning—Ability to logical thinking
- Perceptual speed—Grasp of visual details
- Numerical ability—Performance using numbers
- Word fluency—Speed in use of words
- Memory—Recall verbal details
- Spatial visualization—Ability in perceiving distance and shapes.

Thurstone assembled battery of tests to measure abilities. Thurstone primary mental ability (PMA) is a more popular intelligence test.

JP Guilford (1967)

JP Guilford expanded the concept of multiple components in intelligence. He described human activities in terms of three basics of test categories of mental abilities.

1. Operations (act of thinking)
2. Contents (terms of words, symbols etc.)
3. Products (the ideas we develop, along these categories of mental abilities).

Guilford: Guilford has proposed a three-dimensional theory of intelligence represented by cubical model. The model provides 120 factors of intelligence or primary abilities which is a combination yield of four contents, five operations, and six products. According to Guilford, there are three types of thinking abilities.

1. **Cognition:** The information is gathered and tested by cognitive process.
2. **Production:** Reflects the used information. Production ability may be convergent, i.e. leading toward a single correct answer or divergent, i.e. taking number of directions (answers), any one or more may be right.
3. **Evaluation:** Cognition and production are verified by the ability and determined by evaluation.

Howard Gardner Eight Types of Intelligence (Multiple Intelligence)

In the 1980s and 1990s, psychologist Howard Gardner proposed the idea of not one kind of intelligence but eight, which are relatively independent of one another. These eight types of intelligence are:

1. **Linguistic:** Spoken and written language skills
2. **Logical-mathematical:** Number skills
3. **Musical:** Performance or composition skills
4. **Spatial:** Ability to evaluate and analyze the visual world
5. **Bodily-kinesthetic:** Dance or athletic abilities
6. **Interpersonal:** Skill in understanding and relating to others
7. **Intrapersonal:** Skill in understanding the self
8. **Nature:** Skill in understanding the natural wordlist.

Gardner believes that the above stages dominate by inherited and culture influenced by environment. Critics of the idea of multiple intelligences maintain that these abilities are talents rather than kinds of intelligence.

Robert Sternberg: Triarchic Theory of Intelligence

Psychologist Robert Sternberg defined intelligence as "mental activity directed toward purposive adaptation to, selection and shaping of, real-world environments relevant to one's life." Sternberg explained to get value for intelligence by three basic elements of analyzation, creativity, and practice.

1. Analytical intelligence: This component refers to problem-solving abilities.
2. Creative intelligence: This aspect of intelligence involves the capacity to deal with new situations using past experiences and current skills.
3. Practical intelligence: This element refers to the ability to adapt to a changing environment.

Jean Piaget (Stage Theory of Cognitive Development)

The Swiss psychologist Jean Piaget (1896–1980) proposed theory on four stages of cognitive development. He focused his knowledge through assimilation by (modifying to environment) challenges of mental abilities by adding correction and reducing unusual ones. He also viewed intellectual development as an evolution of cognitive processes understanding the laws of nature and principles of grammar.

Cattell's Theory of General Intelligence

RB Cattell (1971) on the basis of factor analysis divided general factor of intelligence into two parts: Flued intelligence and crystalized intelligence. He focused on determination of innate, biological genetic processes and later acquiring of educational cultural experiences. Both are independent and interrelated to assume person's general intelligence.

Assessment of Intelligence

Alfred Binet (1875–1911) was the first psychologist **(Fig. 3.53)** to devise an intelligence test: Binet and Theodore Siman developed their intelligence scale in 1905. In this method, there is a scale arranged with 30 difficult items. This test is used to measure intelligence based on observation in prescribed topics.

The test was developed by Binet and Simon to identify mentally retarded children in French schools and succeeded in reaching the goal. Subsequently, several English language versions of the test were produced to measure intelligence. Lewis Terman **(Fig. 3.54)** was the first developer of Stanford-Binet scale from Standard University in 1916. Stanford-Binet intelligence scale is popular in measuring intelligence.

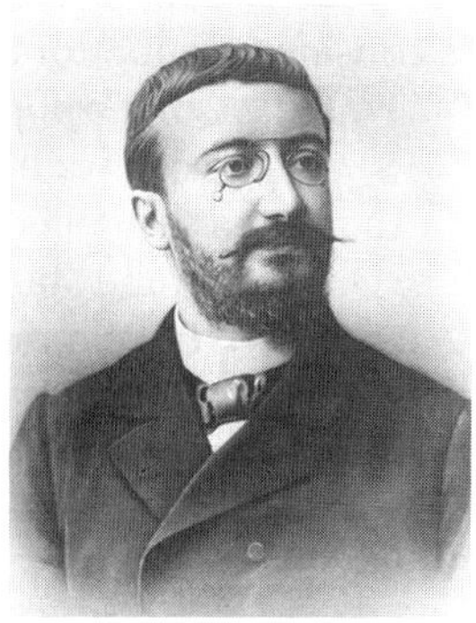

Fig. 3.53: Alfred Binet key developer of Stanford Binet test

Intelligence Quotient

The abbreviation IQ was coined by the psychologist William Stern, a German psychologist and philosopher.

The intelligence quotient is used to know the retarded level of the individual by task performance.

The Stanford-Binet Intelligence Test—In this test, intelligence quotient is measured by the measurement of mental age (the score on the test) divided by chronological age and then multiplied by 100. The test is designed that the average score will always be 100, which means that our mental and chronological ages are equal.

Chronological age (CA)–actual age

Mental age (MA) is determined by score of task performance in a systematic procedure. Cognitive development slows at 16 and then stops at 18, making the calculation of mental age irrelevant. Mental age does not increase steadily life long, but chronological age (original age) increases until death.

Lewis Terman

In the US, Lewis Terman adapted Binet's test for American school children and named the test the Stanford-Binet Test. The following is the formula of Intelligence Quotient (IQ), introduced by William Stern:

$$IQ = \frac{\text{Mental age}}{\text{Chronological age}} \times 100$$

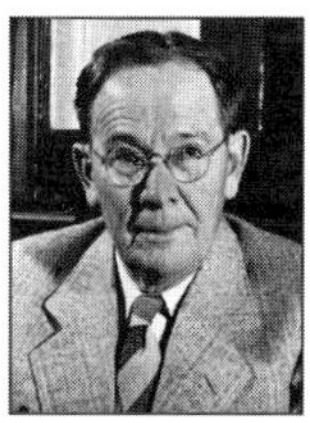

Fig. 3.54: Lewis Terman

Examples

IQ = 100 × MA/CA
MA = 14 years/CA = 10 years (IQ = 140 which means gifted)
MA = 7 years/CA = 10 years (IQ = 70 which means retarded)

The formula for calculating IQ developed by Terman was 100 × MA/CA.

The achievement of scale by an individual is called an intelligence scale. By conducting different IQ tests for the past several years, average IQ on test is 100. An IQ score of 130 or above is considered superior level.

Only 2.2% of the population has an IQ score below 70 (American Psychological Association 2013). A score of 70 or below indicates significant cognitive delays. Mental retardation is caused and accepted as intellectual disability by four subtypes—mild, moderate, severe, and profound. The Diagnostic and Statistical Manual of Psychological Disorders list criteria for each sub-group (APA-2013)). In general, intelligence tests measure a wide variety of human behavior better than any other measure that has been developed.

Wechsler Tests (Table 3.1)

As (WISC-R, 1974) and Wechsler Adult Intelligence Scale WAIS, 1981: These tests are individual tests based on task performance. These are more useful in investigation on brain functioning of humans.

Bhatia's battery of performance is also widely used to measure individual intelligence. This test has subtests, namely, Kohn's Block design test and pad picture construction test.

A comparison between Binet scale and Wechsler scales: Binet scales (1908–1972) are age scales, whereas Weschler's **(Fig. 3.55)** scales are point scales aware of the problem.

Kaufman-Anderson test (KAT) is a group intelligence test which measures intelligence covering knowledge through 12th grade.

The cognitive abilities test is another important group intelligence test.

Development of Intelligence

According to Pinter, the intelligence grows rapidly until 14 years and slows down from 14 to 22 years of age. Ottis expressed that it grows until 18 years.

In the opinion of Terman, students and adults reach the limit of their intelligence growth at the age of 16 years. According to Benet, this limit is reached at the age of 15 years. Thorndike opinion is that it grows until 22 years and it continues up to 45 years of their age in normal individuals.

Table 3.1: WAIS–III

Wechsler Tests IQ Range ("deviation IQ")	*IQ Classification*
130 and above	Very superior
120–129	Superior
110–119	High average
90–109	Average
80–89	Low average
70–79	Borderline
69 and below	Extremely low

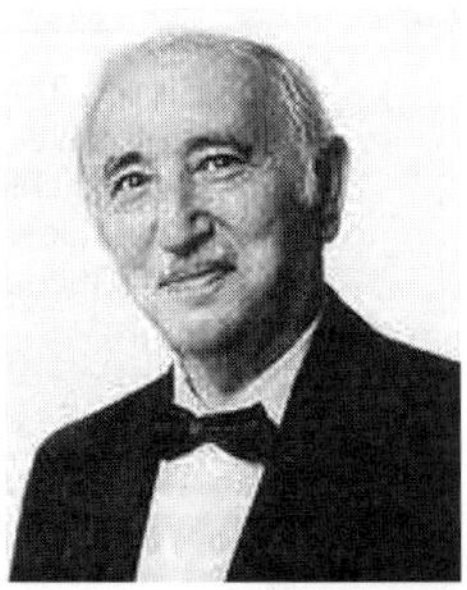

Fig. 3.55: B Wechsler

List of Popular Intelligence Tests

- Stanford-Binet Intelligence Scales
- Wechsler-Adult Intelligence Scale
- Wechsler Intelligence Scale for Children
- Wechsler Primary and Preschool Scale of Intelligence
- Raven's Progressive Matrices (non-verbal test)
- Cattell Culture Fair III
- Thurstone's Primary Mental Abilities
- Multidimensional Aptitude Battery.

These tests also provide information on cultural and biological differences among people.

Types of Intelligence Tests (Fig. 3.56)

Individual tests: The intelligence may differ from one individual to another. The difference occurs by several reasons like heredity and environment, physical and psychological conditions of human beings. These individual tests help to know mental ability by performance of task in each individual separately. These are also helpful to diagnose the differences on human growth by comparing general human being by verbal and nonverbal tests.

Verbal tests, e.g.: Stanford-Binet test: Stanford-Binet test is an individual test. In this test, items are by oral selection. It is a verbal test to know the individual ability on comprehension, reasoning, vocabulary, memory, etc.

Performance tests: Performance tests are useful when the person being tested cannot speak language in cases of deaf or dumb, minimum or minimum educational background.

The test is conducted by picture design, assembling blocks, missing digits to complete, etc. These are non-verbal tests to know the ability of individual intelligence to promote education and performance by using special techniques.

Group Tests: Group tests are mostly used in military and schools to administer with group problems.

Group tests are widely used to recruit people in military and admission in colleges and schools and other employment sector.

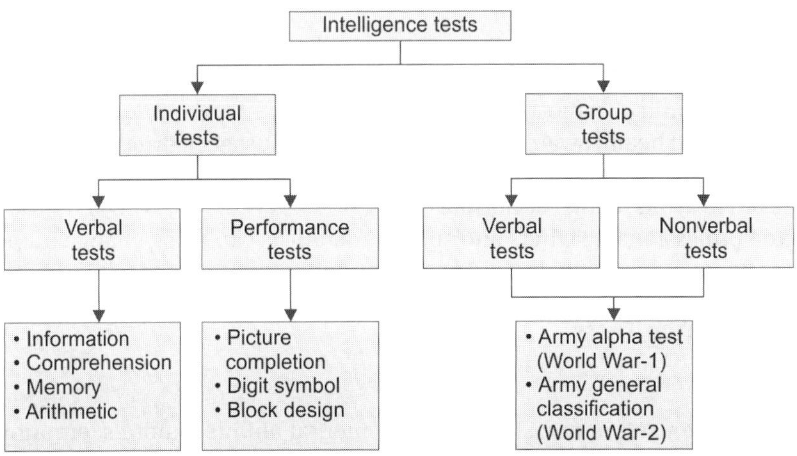

Fig. 3.56: Types of intelligence tests

Army Alpha test in World War 1: The army Alpha test was developed for those who could read. It is emphasized on both verbal abilities and administration.

Army General classification test (developed in world war 2): The Army Beta Test emphasized on the nonverbal abilities and was to be given to those who performed poorly on these Alpha test and were suspected of having language problems.

Teachers and psychologists used these tests to know the levels of intelligence development. Sometimes these are useful to diagnose the mental ability. These are also useful in group therapies of alcoholism, drug addiction, etc.

Group tests were designed as mass testing instruments; they not only permit the simultaneous examination of large groups but they also use simplified instruction and administration procedures, thereby requiring a minimum of training on the part of examiner.

Scores of the group test generally depend on the reading ability. Information obtained by the group test is generally less accurate than the individual tests.

Examples:

- Multidimensional aptitude battery
- The cognitive abilities test
- Scholastic assessment tests.

Individual Differences in Intelligence

Heredity and environment are main causes to get individual on human intelligence.

The genetic factors are powerful in transmitting traits to future generations and inspired by environmental factors in intelligence.

The gender differences are also possible by studies conducted on males and females to know intelligence levels of human traits. But in most cases, no significant difference has been noticed.

Intelligence on cultural differences: Earlier studies in USA which indicated the whites to be a superior race to the blacks have been questioned. Present indications are intelligence not depending on the race or group. Some psychological study on intelligence was influenced by nutritious food, planning, culture, etc.

Causes of Mental Retardation

Most of the psychological studies tell that 25% of all causes of mental retardation are due to physical disorders like birth injuries, using drugs in pregnancy, genetic abnormalities, metabolic disorders, and chromosomal disorders.

The education and health awareness like risk factors on usage of drugs by pregnant women, marital custom within their blood circle, publicity, and free treatment on these are important steps to be taken to avoid mental abnormal births.

Most of the professional teachers and speech therapists can bring change in modification of behavior children in psychological awareness by applying teaching techniques.

Uses of Intelligence Tests

Use for Diagnosis

Intelligence tests are used in measuring certain mental abilities, morals, emotions, general temperament, and ability to work with other people.

The intelligence quotient score is more useful in recognition of intelligence levels of children and adults to diagnose the retardedness of the individual or group.

Educational Sector

To know the ability of the student in selection of different types of professional courses. The results of intelligence tests along with the achievement tests can be successfully used for promotion of students to the next higher grades of classes.

Employment and Business

The different types of intelligence tests are used in recruitment of employees in different organizations, by planning projects to get profits on a particular field by conducting interview or group discussion to assess the intelligence of the individual.

In business, planning and ability are very important to get success or failure in particular area. Sometimes it leads to frustration and even suicide. The intelligence levels are more essential in investing and planning major projects.

Testing of Interest in Music, Dance, or Films

Most of the experts in these fields are using different intelligence tests to assess the individual on particular subjects toward their best future. They are guiding them toward right track.

Intelligence tests are used to judge the learning capacity of an individual by conducting tests.

APTITUDE

Aptitude means ability or a skill or a potential. Intelligence is a measure of general ability of an individual and aptitude is a special ability.

Aptitude: "A person with an aptitude for mathematics is able to learn mathematical skills with relative ease."

Aptitude is either physical or mental process and develops knowledge toward achievement. It may get both by heredity or environment. The musicians may show interest in playing special music instruments by their learning ability and will. It explains that specific aptitude refers to potential in an area whereas general aptitude refers to potential in several fields.

Some children may show special interest in mechanism of toy cars and replacement of parts of the toy; in later days, they plan to become mechanical engineers or automobile engineering, etc. Some political background may create interest to become politicians in future days. It is also a special ability to develop aptitude.

The tests assume that people differ in their special abilities and that these differences can be useful in predicting future achievements.

Freeman (1971) said that "it is a combination of characteristics indicative of an individual's capacity to acquire (with training) some specific knowledge skill, or a set of organized responses, such as the ability to speak a language, to become a musician, to do a mechanical work."

General or multiple aptitude tests are like intelligence tests in that they measure a broad spectrum of abilities of verbal comprehension, general reasoning, numerical operations,

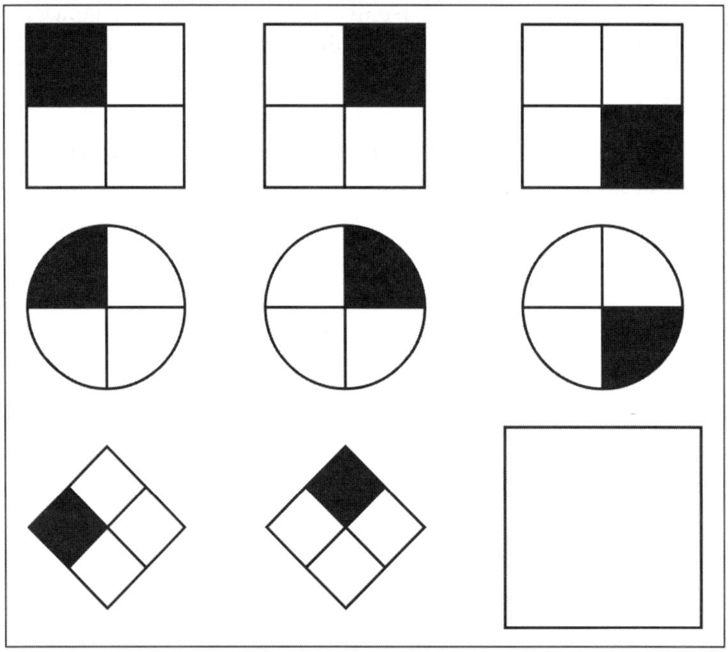

Fig. 3.57: Example of aptitude test

perceptual speed, or mechanical knowledge. The Scholastic Assessment test (SAT) is the example of group test.

Aptitude tests **(Fig. 3.57)** have also been developed to measure special professional values as lawyers, doctors, cricketers, film actors, etc.

In measuring aptitude, the above tests are useful in recruitment of employees into several professions by scrutinizing their skills.

Measures of Aptitudes

Psychologists have developed many tests to measure these aptitudes.

The general learning ability is measured by the test name GATB General Aptitude Test Battery, Differential Aptitude Test (DAT).

Types of Aptitudes

- Sensory aptitude—ability of sense organs vision, auditory, touch, taste, and smell.
- Mechanical aptitude
- Artistic aptitude—expressions on music, sculpture, poetry, designing, painting, dance, photography, acting, etc.
- Professional aptitude—Interest in choosing occupations of teaching, navy, military, legal, pilot, and banks.
- Scholastic aptitude—This aptitude of the scholastic nature includes scientific research, medical, sports, engineering, commercial business fields, etc.

Psychometric Assessment of Cognitive Process

Psychometrics is a field of study concerned with the theory and technique of psychological measurement.

Psychometric: As defined by National Council on Measurement in Education (NCME), psychometrics refers to psychological measurement.

Generally, it refers to the field in psychology and education that is devoted to testing, measurement, assessment, and related activities.

Generally, four types of psychometric tests, numerical reasoning, verbal reasoning, picture analyzation, and judgment tests are more useful in studying different skills and diagnosing the disorders in human behavior.

Numerical reasoning test is useful to assess knowledge in comparing the percentage, proportion of ratio, and rating trends to assess the responses in this type of numerical psychometric test.

Verbal reasoning tests assess skills like true or false or cannot say in statements.

Judgment tests are used to verify the answers and their values and benefits toward their business by using this psychometric test.

Cognitive processes are objective measurement of skills and knowledge, abilities, personality traits, etc. Some psychometric researchers are using construction of qualitative and quantitative methods in assessment. They plan questionnaires, judging, and validation in assessment of personality, attitudes, beliefs, and academic achievement. Another part of the field is concerned with statistical research bearing on measurement theory. Psychometric research involves two major tasks: (i) the construction of instruments and (ii) the development of procedures for measurement. Practitioners are described as psychometricians.

CONCLUSION

The study of cognitive processes is very useful in nursing profession. The study of attention process helps nurses in development of psychological alert toward patient and in diagnosis of disease. The nurse can focus on rehabilitative steps by learning of attention in her academics. All nursing activities require accurate observation and perception. Perceptual knowledge helps the nurse in assessing the critical condition of the patient to prevent the death of the patient. The nurse prompts the other medical team to support the patient in critical condition by her perceptual knowledge. The learning process helps the nurse in understanding and adjusting to manage rapport between patient and nurse toward the treatment. The experience and repetition of the same cases guide the nurse to improve professional knowledge for well-being of the society. The improvement techniques of memory help the nurse in motivating and training the patient to take medicine in time, punctuality in her profession, and in taking care of the patience in her regular practice.

The reasoning and analytical process of thinking levels helps her in success of profession. The study of intelligence and assessment skills are more useful to nurses in understanding mental condition, malfunctioning of brain, causes for low levels of intelligence, etc. The knowledge of aptitude and measuring helps the nurse in development skills in her profession. The nurse can guide the patient and in her working community by using different aptitude tests in her practice.

QUESTIONS

Essay Questions

1. Define attention. Explain determinants of attention.
2. Define perception and explain the principles of perception.
3. Define learning. Explain the theories of learning.
4. What is memory and explain types of memory?
5. Define thinking and discuss the types of thinking.
6. What is intelligence? Discuss the theories of intelligence.
7. Define intelligence. Explain the assessment of intelligence and write the applications of intelligence.
8. Define aptitude. Explain the psychometric assessment of aptitude.
9. What is intelligence? Discuss the development and nature.
10. What is a gifted (mentally superior) child? How will you plan their care and management?

Write Short Notes

1. Span of attention.
2. Factors and control and divert attention.
3. Errors in perception.
4. Illustrate the factors determining perception.
5. Laws of learning.
6. Explain trial and error learning.
7. Conditioning theories of learning.
8. Explain the factors of learning.
9. Stages of memory.
10. Describe the steps of creative thinking.
11. Inductive and deductive reasoning.
12. Distribution of intelligence.
13. Uses of intelligence tests.
14. Psychometric assessment.
15. Name the types of sensory memory.
16. Discuss the memory, retention, and forgetting.
17. Conditioned theories of learning.
18. Factors that control and divert attention.
19. Enlist the characteristics of perception.
20. Differentiate between illusion and hallucination with examples.
21. Alterations in learning that need to improve the quality of nursing.
22. Define thinking and explain the types of thinking.
23. How does the thinking influence the language and communication.
24. Explain the methods of memorizing and describe forgetting.
25. Explain types and process of thinking.
26. Detail the methods of memorizing.

Brief Answers

1. Define span of attention.
2. Internal factors of attention.
3. Alterations in attention.
4. Expand form of LTM and STM.
5. Amnesia and types of amnesia.
6. Formula IQ.
7. Differentiate between mental age and chronological age.
8. Differentiate between incentives and reinforcement.
9. Define transfer of learning.
10. Define amnesia.
11. Enumerate the classification of intelligence.
12. Differentiate between anterograde amnesia and retrograde amnesia.
13. Name the types of sensory memory.
14. Enumerate different types of thinking.
15. Define study habits.
16. Define learner and learning.
17. List the advantages of reinforcement.
18. Define creative thinking.
19. Enumerate types of hallucination.
20. Write the aptitude in the individual differences.
21. List the cognitive process and psychometric assessment.
22. Define the duration and degree of attention.
23. Enumerate the methods of learning.
24. Write the formula for calculating intelligence quotient.

Fill in the Blanks

1. Sensation + ________________ = perception (attention).
2. Ross classification of attention classified into volitional and ________________ attention. (non-volitional)
3. One individual can attend in a given time and at a glance number of letters, digits one can see and reproduce in ________________ attention. (span of)
4. Figure and ground, proximity, similarity, and closer are some of the ________________ of perception. (principles)
5. Illusion and hallucination are ________________ in perception. (errors)
6. Learning is a process of ________________ behavior. (modification)
7. Law of readiness, law of exercise, and law of effect are Thorndike 3 ________________ of leaning. (laws)
8. Pavlov designed an apparatus to measure the quantity of saliva produced in response to food (meat power) in ________________ theory of leaning. (classical conditioned)
9. In ________________ conditioning theory of learning, Skinner conducted his famous experiment by placing a hungry rat in a box called after his name "Skinner box." (operant or instrumental)

10. Observational learning or Social learning initially described by ________________ occurs through observing the behaviors of others and imitating those behaviors, even if there is no reinforcement at the time. (Albert Bandura)
11. In the development process of memory, three stages are encoding, ________________ and retrieval. (Storing)
12. Amnesia may be one of the symptoms of some degenerative brain diseases such as Alzheimer's ________________. (disease)
13. In ________________ type of amnesia, a patient can remember data and events which happened before the injury. (anterograde)
14. Dementia refers to a large class of disorders characterized by the progressive deterioration of thinking ability and memory as the brain becomes ________________. (damaged)
15. Thinking is a cognitive process which involves________________. (perceiving and remembering)
16. The formula for calculating IQ developed by Terman was 100 × ________________ (MA/CA).
17. In Wechsler scale IQ score of normal individual is between 90 and________________ (109).
18. Intelligence is a measure of general ability; aptitude is a ________________ ability. (special)
19. Language, observation and perception, non-verbal behavior, silence listening, and watching are ________________ of communication (tools).
20. Psychometrics is a field of study concerned with the theory and technique of________________ measurement (psychological).

Multiple Choice Questions

1. Involuntary attention can be known as ....
   a. Non-volitional
   b. Volitional
   c. Implicit
2. Following are the external factors which affect attention ....
   a. Interest
   b. Intensity, novelty etc.
   c. Aptitude
3. Perception gives meaning to ....
   a. Hallucination
   b. Illusion
   c. Sensation
4. Perceptual disorder are ....
   a. Illusions and hallucination
   b. Figure and ground
   c. None
5. False in perception is ....
   a. Hallucination
   b. Illusion
   c. None

6. Learning is a process of .... of behavior.
   a. Response
   b. Goal direction
   c. Modification
7. Laws of leaning are summed by ....
   a. Woodworth
   b. Thorndike
   c. None
8. Classical condition is also called ....
   a. Learning by insight
   b. Conditioning
   c. Instrumental conditioning
9. Thinking is a .... mental activity.
   a. Memory
   b. Motivated
   c. None
10. Intelligence measured as ....
    a. Intelligence quotient
    b. Blood investigation
    c. Radiological
11. Chronological age is defined as ....
    a. Mental age
    b. Mental development
    c. Actual age
12. According to Terman's classification of intelligence quotient normal IQ is ....
    a. 91–110
    b. 120
    c. 71–80
13. IQ formula ....
    a. CA/Ma × 100
    b. MA/CA × 100
    c. None

Answers

1. a	2. b	3. c	4. a	5. b	6. c	7. a	8. c	9. b	10. a	11. c	12. b	13. b

4 CHAPTER

Motivation and Emotional Processes

Learning Objectives

- Motivation meaning, concepts, type, theories, motives and behavior, conflict resolution
- Emotions and stress
- Emotion: Definition, components, changes in emotions, theories, emotional adjustment, emotions in health and illness.
- Stress: Stressors, cycle, effect, adaptation cycle, effect, adaptation and coping
- Attitude: Meaning, nature, development, factors affecting, attitudinal change
- Psychometric assessment of emotions and attitudes
- Alterations in emotions
- Applications

MOTIVATION, EMOTION, AND STRESS

Motivation is stimulating person to act in achievement of desirable goal but emotion is expressing the feelings affected by motives and driving toward success or failure. Many psychologists believe that there is a link between motivation, emotions, and stress **(Fig. 4.1)**. Sometimes the failures in desires lead to depression by severe stress.

MOTIVATION: MEANING, CONCEPTS, TYPE, THEORIES, MOTIVES, AND BEHAVIOR, CONFLICT RESOLUTION

Motivation is based on behavior of human beings and animals. Motivation literally means to move, to energize, and to activate. Motivation is an internal force which accelerates a response or behavior. Motivation includes all internal conditions, which begin an activity and sustain it till the goal is achieved.

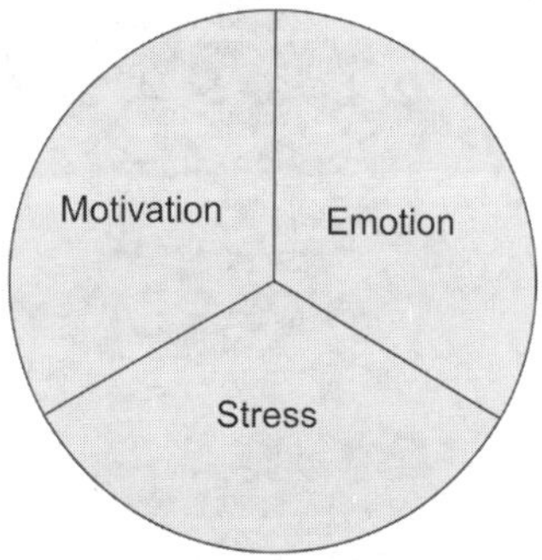

Fig. 4.1: Link of motivation, emotion and stress on human behavior

Motivation is derived from the Latin word "movere" which means "to move," to "energize" or "to activate." Motivation is defined as "conditions" within the organism which arouse, maintain, and direct behavior toward a specific goal. The motivational process reduces tension by fulfilling desires and makes body to normal. The repetition of these processes of motivation can become habit, belief, and desire in routine life. It acts to the needs of the individual.

Some Introductory Psychology books define the field of motivation as the study of goal-directed behavior.

Definition

Morgan and King (1975): "Motivation refers to the states within a person or animal that drives behavior toward some goals."

Underwood (1968): "Motivation means the classes of operations used to produce and measure changes in performance and changes in energy output." Motivation is defined as "conditions within the organism which abuse, maintain, and direct behavior toward a specific goal.

Carol (1969): A need gives rise to one or more motives. A motive is rather specific process, which has been learned. It is directed toward a goal.

Components of Motivation

The four components of motivation **(Fig. 4.2)** are need, drive, response, and goal.

Drive: A drive is an aroused state resulting from needs of body. It needs energy to perform task both physical and psychological satisfaction of needs. The individual seeks to reduce this drive by active process for satisfaction of needs.

Goal or incentive: The goal makes person to struggle for success. The fulfillment of desires is difficult without proper preparation or goal for performance of task. The planning procedure drives the individual in planning of every performance. Success is reaching destination and planned schedule is possible by only planning of goal or incentive in human behavioral processes.

It arouses the organism toward success of achievement. A goal refers to some substance, objects, or environment condition capable of reducing to temporary elimination of complex and internal conditions which are initiated by action.

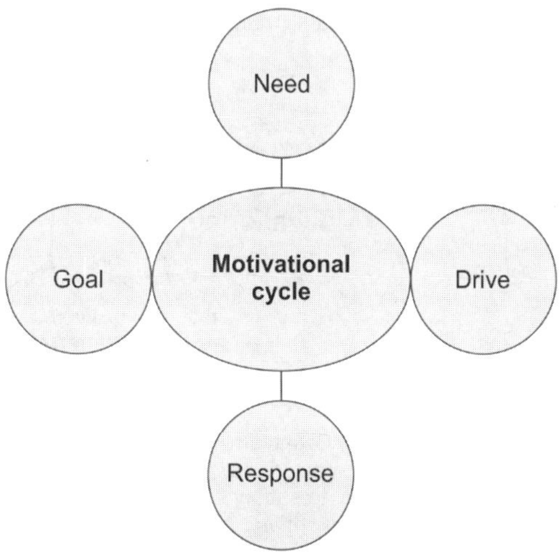

Fig. 4.2: Components of motivation

The goal is a gift and provides psychological pleasure and leads to be energetic in performing tasks. An incentive refers to the motivational value of reinforced. Without incentive motivation cannot be fulfilled.

Needs

Needs are general desires based on behavior. The needs are the priorities for physical and psychological well-being of individual. Every individual struggles for existence. The human beings are satisfied by both biological and psychological needs in achieving goals. Needs make the person to face challenges or risks in fulfilling of desires of individuals or groups. Necessity makes the person to adjust difficult circumstances in achievement of success in day-to-day life.

Homeostasis: Claude Bernard coined the word "homeostasis" to explain the stability of the inner environment or physiological equilibrium. This process is automatic in nature and the maintenance of balance they attain is referred to homeostasis. Primary motives are essential for survival. A motive activates the individual and drives to satisfy the desires and develops interest for specific behavior.

Response: Response is motivated behavior. Motives are the dynamics of human behavior. Responsibility is not a simple process in managing the circumstances of human life. Responsibility leads the person for challenges in achievement of success. In acceptance of response is essential in every moment of life. Most of the people analyze the process in proper direction which gives self-satisfaction.

Motivational Cycle

Motivation cycle is based on components (drives, need, goal, and response) and types of both primary and secondary motives **(Fig. 4.3)**.

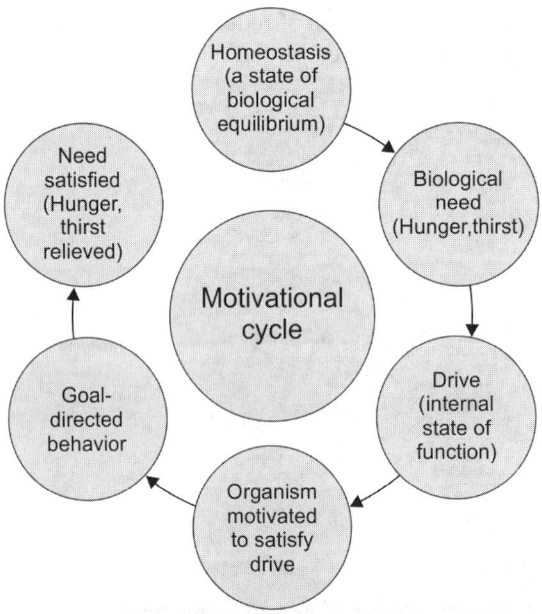

Fig. 4.3: Motivational cycle

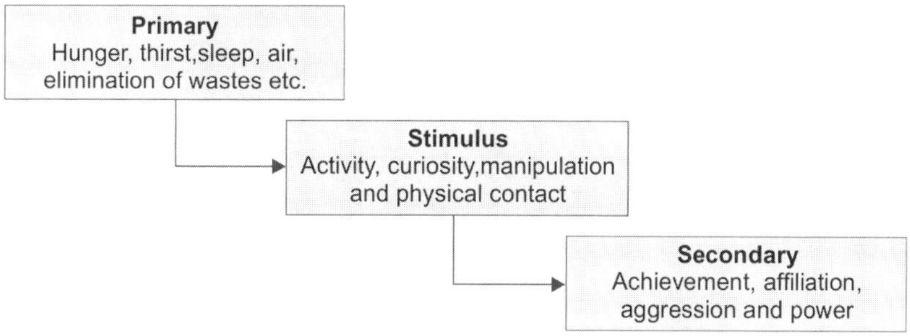

Fig. 4.4: Types of motives

Types of Motives (Fig. 4.4)

Primary Motives

These are physiological motives and unlearned motives. In these motives, hunger, sex, thirst, oxygen, rest, and sleep are included. The fulfillment of these primary motives makes the individual to avoid discomfort and provides relief from pain, activity, and in elimination of needs. It creates comfortable life to cope up social circumstances for both physical and mental activities in day-to-day life. Dissatisfaction of drives leads to changes in human behavior like irritation, anger, and restlessness. The fulfilment of primary motives leads to good health. Sufficient food, water, sleep, and oxygen are more essential for life span expansion.

Biological Motivation and Homeostasis

Biological motives are also called physiological motives. These motives are essential for the survival of the organism. The body always tends to maintain a state of equilibrium called "Homeostasis" in many of its internal physiological processes. The nutritious food, sufficient fluids, and level of temperature are important features to maintain homeostasis.

Hunger Drive

This is one of the dominant drives that help for the proper functioning of human body. If the intake of food is irregular, it leads to certain biochemical changes in the tissues of the body causing stomach pain—an indication of contraction of stomach muscles due to pain or discomfort.

Excess eating, quality of food, and speed in eating are leading complications in human digestive system. The fulfillment of hunger drive **(Fig. 4.5)** brings back the body into normal physiological balance or homeostasis. The intake of food in regular process is the only solution to manage this hunger drive. The nutrient values in food are also one of the important aspects to maintain healthy levels of physical health.

The food, including carbohydrates and fats, after digestion changes into glucose and amino acids mixed into blood and supplies to all parts of body. It gives energy for best functioning of body. According to the lady researcher, Doctor Christine Y Lee, a gastroenterologist, hunger makes the person not only angry but also has effects on differences in human behavior. After usage of energy on these activities, the glucose levels become low and continuation leads to hormonal changes developed in human body. It causes anger, lack of energy, drowsiness, lack of attention, loss of memory, etc.

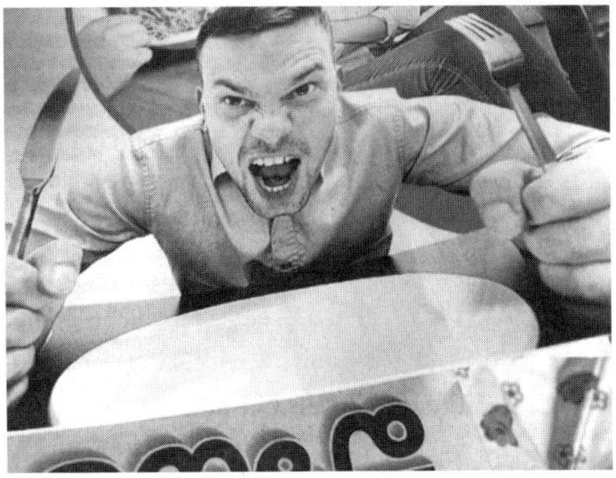

Fig. 4.5: Facial expressions in human body by hunger drive leads to anger

The food is more essential in human life. Unequal intake levels of food cause ill-health and indigestion. The biochemical processes get their energy from them.

Thirst Drive

Satisfying of the thirst helps in balancing of human body temperature, levels of digestion, and in elimination of wastes. These functions occur automatically in our body. The intake of fluids like water and juice can manage hunger drive for some more hours. The longevity of intake of only fluids without solids results in loss of energy and affects body activities for a long duration of life. Quality and quantity are more important points in digestion. Sometimes eating oily or fried solid items causes excessive thirst. The fluids are essential for digestion of solids. The decrease of water level in the body causes thirst drive and dehydration. The water level is low in the mouth; it becomes dry and affects our speech.

Experiments by psychologists expressed that wetness is not enough to satisfy the thirst drive.

Respiratory Drive

This drive for air and oxygen helps in breathing. People cannot survive with insufficient supply of oxygen or air in human body. The slow supply of oxygen or air causes suffocation, weakness, giddiness, and some other changes for improper functioning of every part of human body. It creates more physical and psychological disturbance in management of body function. Sometimes, with irregularities in respiration, humans cannot survive for a long life. If the individual faces difficulty in breathing for a long period, it can lead to death. The respiratory drive is very important than other primary motives. Breathing problem affects sleep and rest. It leads to malfunction of brain. These are major causes of damage in brain function. Oxygen is necessary in purification of blood. Our body needs oxygen continuously. The supply of oxygen is blocked or disturbed in blood circulation which causes heart attack, asthma, etc.

Sleep Drive

Sleep drive is one of the important aspects in balancing all the drives of human body. Lack of sleep disturbs daily activities by lapse of memory and concentration and discomfort to perform day-to-day activities. The lack of sleep leads to physical weakness, loss of appetite etc. It is continued for a long duration which causes depression, anxiety disorders, etc. Individual loses interest in social relations and prefers loneliness. The human body needs rest by good sleep. Enough sleep improves memory and energizes physical activities. These help to prolong human life span. Sometimes it is very difficult to control sleep after long duration of physical strain. The satisfaction of the sleep drive helps to free from psychological and physical tiredness. Thus, the sleep drive has an active role in mind and body function. Enough sleep helps in good thinking power and concentration. It decreases confusion status, droopy eyelids, muscle tremors, etc.

Drive Elimination of Waste

Satisfaction of hunger and thirst drive has more influence on elimination of wastes from our body. The proper function of body organs depends on the process of elimination of wastes. The physical changes in body depend on elimination of wastes. Excessive intake of food and water has excessive effects on digestion like diarrhea and other body functional changes in physical health. When the bladder or intestine becomes distended with waste material, they cause pressure and discomfort. The person may feel difficult to sleep, lose temperament, lack of concentration, irritability, and other changes in human behavior due to irregularity of elimination of waste.

Sex drive is considered a biological drive and is dependent on physiological conditions of human personality. The sex drive comes from nervous tension and by sex hormones. Its control and acceptance is connected to moral, cultural, and civil codes of law of the society. The sex drive can be managed by engaging mind on other interested activities of the individual. The person feels difficulty in changing mood from sex drive to another goal.

The fulfillment of sex drive depends on cultural and traditional circumstances of the individual who belongs to different societies. We have to sublimate this drive by engaging ourselves with art and painting; creativity of thoughts is an important skill in diversion of sex drive. This is a biological motive, which arises in the organism as a result of secretion of sex hormones. Sex need is not essential for the survival of the individual, but it is essential for the survival of the species.

Marriage is an important custom in Indian families. Applying restrictions is very important in fulfilling sexual desires in Indian families. In Indian society, family is more valuable and to future generation on values of sex and implementation. The wrong track in fulfilling sexual drive is severely punishable by law and order of society and culture. In fulfillment of sex drive, some limitations are considerable in human beings.

Secondary Motives/Social Motives or Learned Motives

Primary motives are more essential than the secondary motives. The secondary motives are fulfilled by hard work, desires, and learning processes. These secondary motives linked with one's socio-psychological need are known as secondary or psychological motives.

Physiological motives are common in both human beings and animals. The above discussed motives pertain to both animals and human beings. The social motives are found only in human beings by result of pressures, competition, and of social interactions in human growth and development. The strength is also a powerful weapon in achieving success of power and status in all societal life. Social motive is different from one individual to another.

Cognitive Theories

Cognitive theories define motivation in terms of how people think about situations. Cognitive theories of motivation include goal-setting theory and expectancy theory.

Social motives are recognized by psychologists. Social motives are also called as learned or secondary motives.

Influence of Human Behavior on Theories of Motivation

Most of the motivational theories are linked on social cognition, humanistic behavior, psychoanalysis, and learning **(Fig. 4.6)**.

Theories of cognitive process and social interactions influence human behavior in achieving the physical and biological needs of the individuals and groups.

Goal-setting theory is based on the notion that individuals sometimes have a drive to reach a clearly defined end state. Often, this end state is a reward in itself.

An ideal goal should present a situation where the time between the initiation of behavior and the end state is close.

Behaviorist Theories

Incentive theory is based on behaviorist learning theories proposed by Thorndike, Pavlov, Watson, and BF Skinner. The incentive theory suggests that people are motivated to do things because of external rewards.

Classical conditioning is understood as responses caused by imposed conditions to train in learning by application of physical stimuli.

Behavior is punished or reinforced to modify the behavior and trained by choosing the correct direction by several sittings for perfectness with reward and punishment by process. The various mechanisms of operant conditioning help to learn in searching of new path with the help of instruments by different trials in modification of behavior. Social learning is the modification behavior that helps to understand social conditions in changing attitudes toward the benefit of the process.

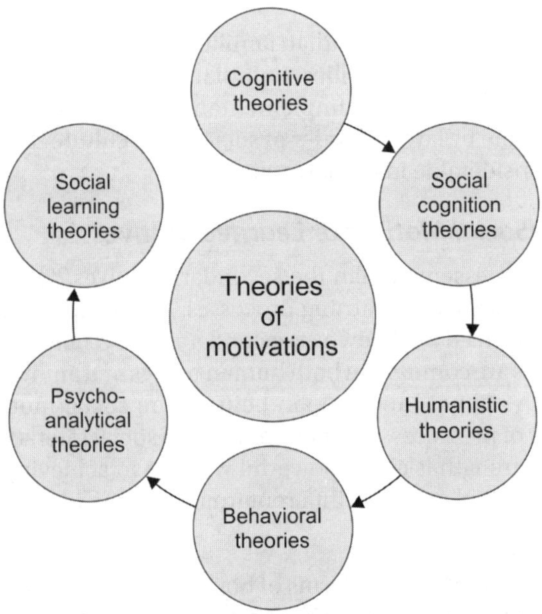

Fig. 4.6: Theories of motivational influences

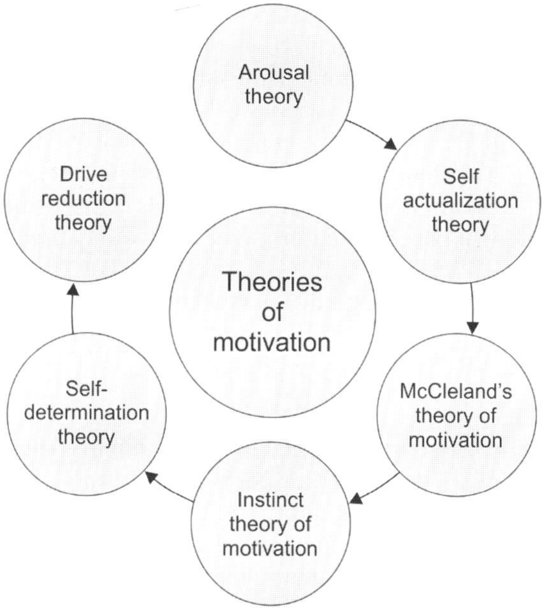

Fig. 4.7: Theories of motivation

Theories of Motivation

Psychologists have proposed some different ways of thinking for arousal of motivation either internal (intrinsic) or external (extrinsic). Intrinsic motivation is natural. It refers to enjoyment and self-satisfaction. Extrinsic motivation is unnatural to obtain reward or outcome. It depends on external factors by performance of tasks to avoid punishment. Some motivational theories **(Fig. 4.7)** are given below:

- McClelland's theory of motivation
- Drive reduction theory of motivation (push theory of motivation)
- Self-actualization theory of motivation, Maslow's theory of motivation
- Arousal theory of motivation
- Instinct theory of motivation (Pull theory of motivation).

McClelland's Theory

McClelland's theory explains that human needs are acquired and shaped by one's life experiences. Most of these needs can be classified as: 1. Achievement, 2. Affiliation, and 3. Power **(Fig. 4.8)**.

McClelland's theory explains that individuals may differ in the degrees of these on behavior.

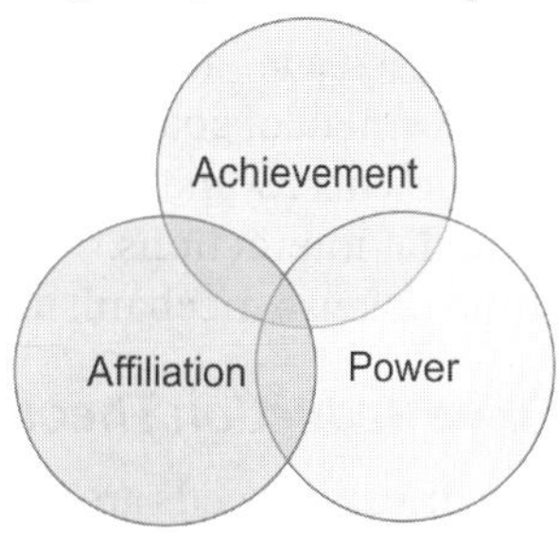

Fig. 4.8: Basics of McClelland's theory of motivation

Achievement

Achievement is depending on goal of the individual and results of its success. Success of achievement is caused by performance of tasks by crossing many obstacles. People may suffer in reaching destination in a satisfied manner. McClelland found that some are good in achievement without failures. They will take personal responsibility in achievement. Some of parents may guide their children in decision-making toward success in it. It helps them to develop achievement motivation in their future. Even they may learn to tolerate some of the failures by lack of achievement in reaching their goal. People are motivated by achievement work very effectively either alone or with other high achievers. They will utilize all their efforts in fulfillment of the desires. People high in this need are characterized by a tendency to seek challenges and high degree of independence. The individual monitors progress and development in all levels of performance.

Achievement motivation is based on performance motive and directed toward performance of personality.

Achievement motivation is an integrative perspective based on harmonious relationship with other people. It is based on motivational performance; results from broad components of personality are directed toward success in reaching goal.

Affiliation

Affiliation depends on coordination of people in leading life in society. Man cannot lead life alone. Man is a social animal. The major task performance is possible only by group process of association, cooperation, and adjustment. The purpose of the group is achievement of goal. People learn all these with the help of social agencies, family, school, neighborhood, religion, and state. Some people are facing problems by lack of adjustment in social relations by competition, conflicts, and isolation.

The need to be with other people is referred as affiliation need. In affiliation, individuals prefer to work and it provides significant personal interaction. People motivated by affiliation of work help best in group environment.

Power

Power motive directs the behavior of dictators, gang leaders, and the builders. A person's need for power is classified into personal and institutional. Social power is defined as the ability or capacity of a person to produce intended effect on the behavior or emotions of other people. Personally, the member who tries to achieve power chooses specific goals and performs tasks to get success in it. If he fails in achieving, choose another method to get success. The power motive is an authoritative and dominating role in social relations and interactions in group.

In organizational and institutional matters, the power motive is more useful to people in interpretation of objects or goals with competitive spirit. It creates an inspiration move toward success in future projects. Those with a high need for power work best when they are in charge. They will give more importance in competing seniority and other rules and regulations of institutions. The power motivators enjoy all these toward success in reaching their goal by task performance.

Aggression, an external behavior that results in losing temperament, causes failures in achievement of goals. It is both verbal and nonverbal communication reaction by fear, anxiety, and violence. Sometimes the power motive is so harmful and an influence for criminal activities in social interactions. The symptoms of aggressive motives can be modified behavior using some defense mechanisms or mental mechanisms.

Drive Reduction Theory (Push Theory of Motivation)

The drives or needs are internal states of arousal or tensions which must be reduced. So, when we experience a drive, we are motivated to reduce this state of tension and pursue actions that will lead to a drive reduction (reduce the state of tension).

Drive theory was developed by Clark Leonard Hull in 1943. Clark Hull **(Fig. 4.9)** was the behaviorist who developed the drive-reduction theory of motivation **(Fig. 4.10)**.

According Hull 1951—When the instinct theory of motivation failed, it was replaced by drive-reduction theory. Physiological need creates an aroused tension state (a drive) that motivated an organism to satisfy the need.

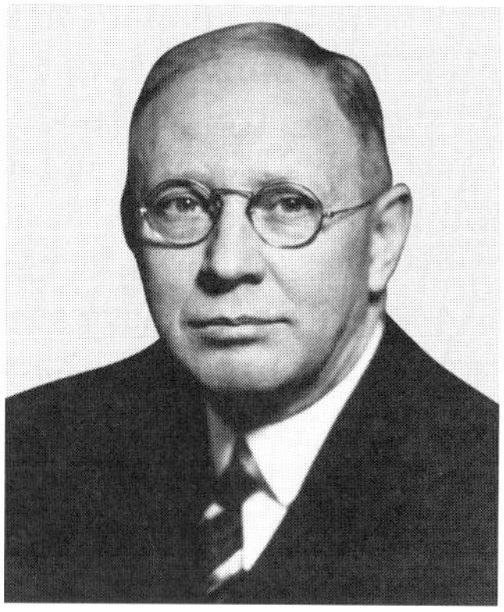

Fig. 4.9: Clark Hull

Upon satisfying a drive, the drive's strength is reduced. The theory became well known in the 1940s and 1950s. Many of the motivational theories that arose during the 1950s and 1960s were either based on Hull's original theory or were focused on providing alternatives to the drive-reduction theory, including Abraham Maslow's hierarchy of needs, which emerged as an alternative to Hull's approach.

According to this theory, a person might be motivated to drink glass of water in order to reduce the internal state of thirst. This theory is useful in explaining behaviors that have strong biological component such as hunger or thirst.

Drive theories must be described as push theories of motivation. Behavior is pushed toward goals by driving states within person.

Motivation may exist without a drive arousal. For example, humans do not like to eat food when there is no hunger motive.

Drive reduction theory grows out of the concept that people have certain biological drives, such as hunger and thirst.

For example, when preparing food, the drive model appears to be compatible with sensations of rising hunger as the food is prepared and disappearance of hunger drive by consuming sufficient food. It decreases interest by success in reaching goal.

According to drive theory of motivation, people are motivated to take certain actions in order to reduce the internal tensions. For example, we might be motivated to drink glass of water in order to reduce the internal state of thirst.

The problem with drive theory of motivation is that this behavior is not always motivated purely by physiological needs. For example, some people fulfill their desires as routine. But they cannot enjoy like others who fulfilled their desire by hunger drive. The meaningful difference is in differentiating these fulfillment drives.

Humanistic Theory by Abraham Maslow and Carl Roger

Maslow Heirarchy Theory

Maslow's theory is one of the most widely discussed theories of motivation. Abraham Maslow believed that man is good in nature by birth and unsatisfaction of these desires move toward the growth of inner drive to satisfy. It needs hierarchy system, devised by Maslow (1954), which is a commonly used scheme for classifying human motives.

Need (e.g. for food, water) → Drive (hunger, thirst) → Drive-reducing behavior (eating, drinking)

Fig. 4.10: Drive reduction theory—Hull 1951

The American motivation psychologist Abraham H Maslow developed the hierarchy of needs consisting of five hierarchic classes. According to Maslow, people are motivating toward un-satisfaction of their needs.

Maslow's hierarchy of needs theory explains that the needs and desires may influence to satisfy the changes in behavior toward achievement of individual goals.

Maslow's hierarchy of needs theory can be summarized as follows:

Human beings have some desires and in fulfilling these they try to do hard work and concentrate toward the success. These influence behavioral changes in human's life. The person gives priority to needs in fulfilling them in order. The least priority also depends on necessity of it in his life. Unfulfilled desires will affect the progress of the hierarchy and lower the psychological health of the person.

Maslow's Theory of Self-actualization

Abraham Maslow in 1954 stated that human needs tend to arrange themselves in hierarchies of self-actualization. Each need appears by depending on another need. These physiological needs are more essential for survival of human beings.

The individual may feel difficulty in adjustment leads to dissatisfaction of both physiological and psychological pleasures.

Maslow's Hierarchy of Needs

The theme of this theory is "human motivation and includes Abraham Maslow's **(Fig. 4.11)** hierarchy of needs and Herzberg's two-factor theory." Maslow's theory is one of the most widely discussed theories of motivation. The hierarchy system, devised by Maslow (1954), is a commonly used scheme for classifying human motives.

- Physiological—Hunger, thirst, sleep, rest, etc.
- Safety—Shelter, security, and health
- Social—Good social relations, love, and friendship
- Self-esteem/recognition/achievement
- Self-actualization—achievement.

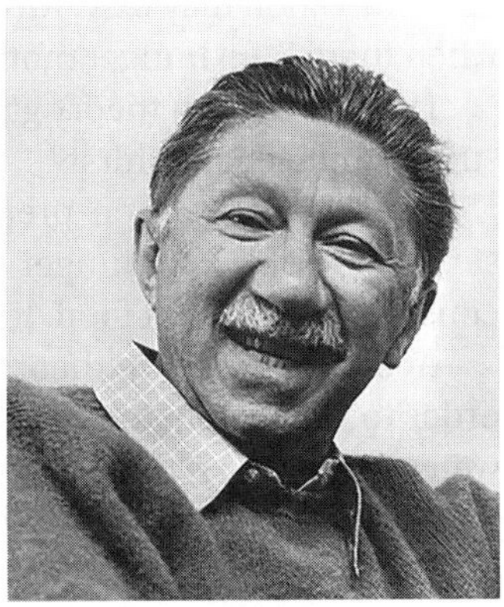

Fig. 4.11: Abraham Harold Maslow

Abraham H Maslow developed the hierarchy of needs consisting of five hierarchic classes **(Fig. 4.12)**.

- **Physiological**: Abraham gave priority for primary needs in his hierarchy motivational theory which include food, water, and shelter. These are basic needs for individuals in common life. If the physiological needs are not fulfilled in time, it leads to some other problems of sickness, mood disorders, irritation, loss of appetite, sleeplessness, etc.
- **Safety and security:** These are social motives to survive in comfortable life. It is also necessary to manage healthy life by fulfillment of basic needs of human beings. Safety refers to shelter and protection of both the physical and social conditions of human life. It gives pleasure to lead a comfortable life for a long duration. It also suggests that love and attention prolongs the human life span not only in individuals but also in group. As a result, they seek out stable lives with careers, homes, insurance, etc.
- **Psychological happiness**: In social interaction, the individual faces different complicated situations and feels discomfort for survival. There is need of love and attention from different directions like family, friends, and society to lead comfortable and happy life. It has

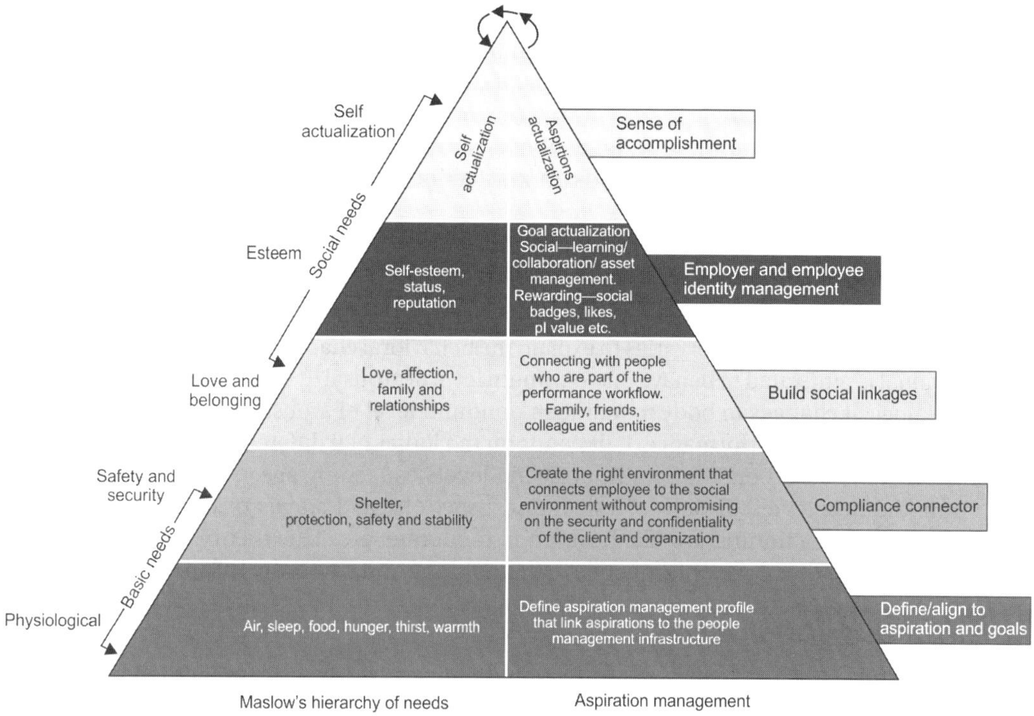

Fig. 4.12: Maslow's pyramid

been shown, in Maslow's theory, that not only physical well-being but also psychological happiness is a need of hierarchy.

- **Esteem:** Person gets esteem from other human beings. People need reciprocity in fulfilling their day-to-day needs. Every human being depends on each other to fulfill desires by using some techniques, power, and authority in different ways of leading life. The satisfaction of necessities creates self-confidence in human life. Dissatisfaction leads to conflicts, depressions, and frustration. Its extremes lead to mental illness. They work hard and face struggles in achievement of esteem and status. It is not an ending process and continues till end of their lives.
- **Self-actualization**: This is very difficult to reaching. According to Maslow, self-actualization is highest human motive. Achieving these stages depends on hard work, talent, and intelligence of humans. The characteristics are differentiated by reality oriented, confidential, novelty, humorous, and creative mind. Maslow framed all these in self-actualization.

Maslow explained that these basic requirements build upon the first step in the pyramid:

The defects of physiological drive may develop several symptoms or disorders in body functioning. For example, lack of intake of food in time leads to disturbance and cooperation for physical activation. Lack of eating leads to sleepless nights and influences irritation and mood disorders.

Subsequently, we have the second level, which awakens a need for security.

After securing those two levels, the motives shift to the social sphere, the third level.

Psychological requirements comprise the fourth level, while the top of the hierarchy consists of self-realization and self-actualization.

Maslow's hierarchy of needs theory can be summarized as follows:

The desires of human beings influence their behavior by arranging in order to get success one by one and it is called hierarchy of needs. It depends on the demands of the individual providing safety and security.

The person advances to the next level of needs only after the lower level need is at least minimally satisfied. The progress depends on satisfaction of desires and provides pleasure and improves psychological well-being.

Arousal Theory of Motivation

The arousal theory suggests that people take certain actions to either increase or decrease levels of arousal **(Fig. 4.13)**. Arousal theory tries to explain the behavioral changes toward process of action. The individual is motivated to behave into optimum level of arousal. It also tries to raise emotional and physiological changes in body to maintain optimum level of arousal. People may reduce or increase depending on performance. It depends on the individual differences in activities.

This theory is based on changes in arousing levels caused by age, gender, brain growth, and strengthening levels of both physical and psychological stages of human being. The performances of functioning are like best, poor, moderate, etc. This theory explains that the capacity of some of the old people is active in their old age and some are dull in their young age.

Instinct Theory of Motivation

According to the Instinct Theory of Motivation, behavior is driven by unlearned or primary motives. Instincts play a major role in basic necessities and their fulfillment. Many of the theories of motivation are similar, except for the amount of emphasis on evolution. Some species are migrating to other areas by choosing suitable climatic conditions. It is an inborn behavior. William James created a list of human instincts like love and attachment, play, guilty, anger, and fear. These are main objectives to motivate human life. These inspire human in improvement of social relations in managing human interactions followed by old generation to new. People are choosing good environment in satisfaction of their desires in modern society. By instincts, they are motivated to learn in search of new methods by following the path of old customs and traditions. They are working hard toward the success of utilization, both nature and nurture.

By the 1920s, instinct theories were pushed aside in favor of other motivational theories; the contemporary evolutionary psychologists are studying the influence of genetics and heredity on human behavior even today.

William McDougal (1908)—influential theorist, who viewed instincts as behavior patterns.

This theory, inspired by Charles Darwin, argues that in the last 15 million years, the human species have evolved socially as well as physically.

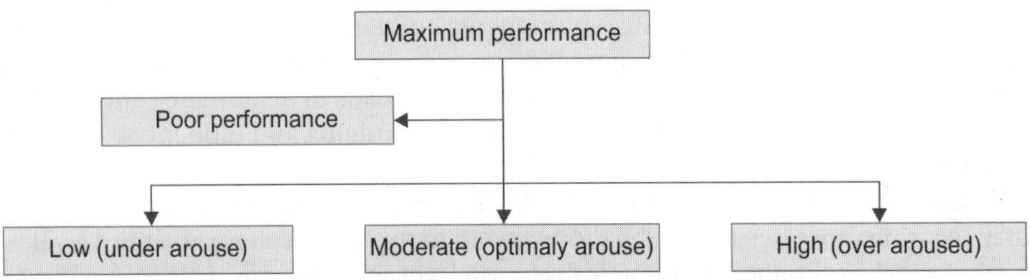

Fig. 4.13: Arousal theory

Most of the modern generations are very serious in planning and selecting areas in development and in creation of new methods in fulfillment of their desires.

The Incentive Theory of Motivation (Pull Theory of Motivation)

Incentive theory is based on behaviorist learning theories by Thorndike, Pavlov, JB Watson, and BF Skinner. It is an external goal-oriented motivational behavior. It pulls to some direction by influencing in performance. For example, players are motivated by the incentive of good score in competing with other teams in sports and games.

The incentive theory suggests that people are motivated to do things because of external rewards. Behavioral learning concepts such as association and reinforcement play an important role in this theory of motivation. Incentive theories are pull theories while drive theories are push theories of motivation. Both are inter-related by forcing behavior in achieving rewards.

The incentive theory has some similarities of BF Skinner behavior modification. Reinforcement strengthens a behavior while punishment weakens it.

Conflicts

Conflicts—stressful condition that occurs when a person must choose between contradictory needs, desires, motives, or demands.

The word conflict has been derived from a Latin word "Conflicts" which means "strike two things at the same time".

According to **Colomn** "A conflict is the anticipated frustration entailed in the choice of either alternative". Conflicts occur in the individual when more than one, equally powerful desires or motives present at the same time, pressurize for immediate satisfaction.

According to **Erik Erikson's** theory of psychosocial development, a conflict is a turning quality. Sometimes referred to as a psychosocial crisis, this can be a time of both vulnerability and strength, as the individual works toward success or failure.

Douglas and Holland: "Conflict means a painful emotional state, which results from a tension between opposed and contradictory wishes".

Types of Conflicts

- **Approach-approach conflict (Fig. 4.14):** This type of conflict occurs between two positive goals or two opposed beliefs that are equally attractive at the same time in decision-making. Person must choose between two desires and outcomes. In this type of conflict, individual will have two desires with positive valence which are equally powerful.

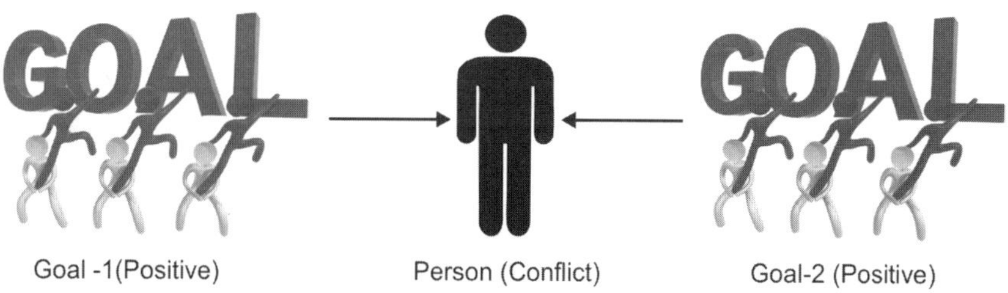

Fig. 4.14: Approach-approach conflict

For example, a person has two favorite programs at the same time, to participate in a function of a friend or attend a close family member function.

Such conflicts are not so harmful, because after selecting one, the other one automatically subsides or loses its importance to him. But in some situation, choice will be very difficult. For example, a girl has to choose either loving parents or a boy-friend for intercaste marriage.

- **Avoidance-avoidance conflict (Fig. 4.15):** It involves two negative goals and the individual is forced to choose one. These types of conflicts are very difficult to resolve tension. Some people cannot continue in employment on one side and another side, they cannot lead life by losing the source of income.

  The individual is caught between two repelling threats, fears, or situations. They cannot choose either of them or may try to escape from the field itself. But the consequences of the escape may also be harmful.
- **Approach-avoidance conflict (Fig. 4.16):** It occurs in two goals, one is attractive and another one has unattractive features. This is also a most complex conflict and very difficult to resolve. Because in this type of conflict, a person is both attracted and repelled by the same goal object.

  Attraction of the goal and inability to approach it lead to frustration and tension.

  For example, a person is approaching to accept a job offer, because the salary is attractive—but at the same time, the type of work is risky to continue for long duration.
- **Multiple approach-avoidance conflicts (Fig. 4.17)**: We must choose between two or more things; some are desirable and undesirable features. Some of the situations in life we come across will involve both positive and negative situations of multiple nature. Suppose a woman is engaged to be married. She may think that marriage gives security and sharing life with life partner is also another attraction which is a positive goal. Another negative thought is connected to neglect of job or career which provides financial assistance in life. In all these situations, conflicts are called as multiple approach-avoidance conflicts. The resolution of this conflict depends upon both situations.

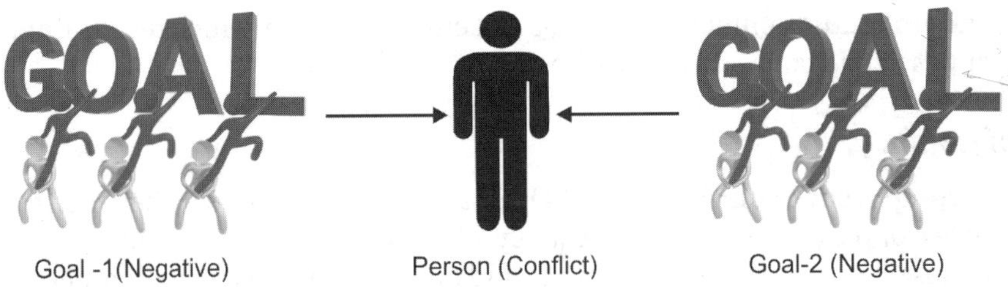

Fig. 4.15: Avoidance-avoidance conflict

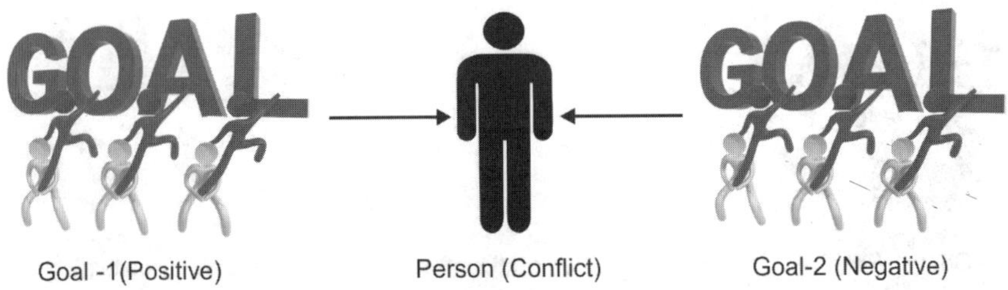

Fig. 4.16: Approach-avoidance conflict

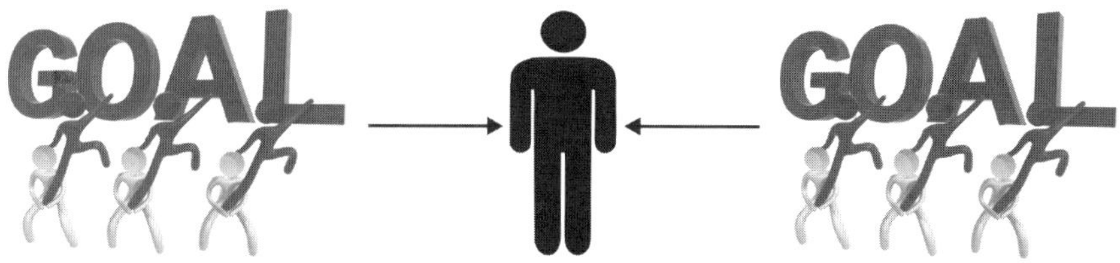

Goal -1(Positive-Negative) Person (Conflict) Goal-2 (Positive-Negative)

Fig. 4.17: Multiple approach-avoidance conflict

Frustrations and Conflicts

Motivation is an internal urge to act toward a particular goal. When motives are hindered or blocked, frustrations and conflicts occur.

Frustration: Frustration is a common emotional response to opposition and is the antithesis of satisfaction.

Good, Carter V: The word frustration has been derived from a Latin word "Frustra" meaning "Obstruct." Frustration refers to the blocking of behavior directed toward the goal. Frustration means emotional tension resulting from the blocking of desire or need.

Frustration is a negative feeling when individual is prevented from reaching the goal. For example, an unemployed may get more expectation by completing his education. The person may get frustrated by disappointment of not succeeding in gaining job for a long period. Frustration occurs when an individual is unable to reach his destination by crossing barriers in both personal and social life.

Resolution of Conflicts

Conflicts give rise to a lot of tension in the individual; he becomes completely disturbed. Tension continues until getting of solution to the conflicted situations.

The conflicts may arise from frustrations, competing roles, or goals having positive or negative goals. Frustration extremes lead to mental ill-health of the individual life. It is very difficult to rebuilt mental hygiene. It is necessary to resolve them as quickly as possible.

The clash between the urges, desires, and motives may go on without being fully aware of it. Conflict resolution depends upon the type of conflict. The double approach conflict may be easily resolved by satisfying one goal first which is more important than the other; for instance, a student attending the class first, then going for food even if hungry.

Interpersonal conflicts: Interpersonal conflict is caused between individuals. Sigmund Freud describes it as a conflict between the forces of the id, the ego, and the super ego, the three dynamics of one's personality. Many of our wants raised by Id may not be socially acceptable. Such wants are objected by the Ego and the Super ego. Hence, these are repressed to unconscious.

Our internal conflict may be conscious or unconscious. The unconscious levels are responsible for mental disorders.

Intrapersonal conflicts: This conflict is resolved by giving up one of the goals. Obviously, approach-approach conflict does not generate much anxiety, because the individual is not going to lose much.

EMOTION

Emotion is a complex, subjective experience accompanied by biological and behavioral changes. Emotion involves feeling, thinking, activation of the nervous system, physiological changes, and behavioral changes such as facial expressions.

An emotion is a complex psychological state that involves three distinct components, a subjective experience, physiological experience, and behavioral or expressive response.

In understanding of emotions, the researchers have tried to identify and classify the different types of emotions. In 1972, psychologist Paul Eckman suggested that there are mainly six basic emotions: fear, surprise, anger, happiness, and sadness. Later he added some more including embarrassment, excitement, contempt, shame, pride, satisfaction, and amusement.

During the 1980s, Robert Plutchik introduced another emotion classification system known as the "wheel of emotions." Plutchik suggested that there are eight primary emotional dimensions: happiness vs. sadness, anger vs. fear, trust vs. disgust, and surprise vs. anticipation.

Definition

The term emotion is derived from the Latin verb "emovere" which means stir up, agitate, disturb, or move.

Woodworth 1945: Emotion is "moved" or "stirred" up state of an organism. It is stirred up state of feeling that is the way it appears to the individual himself. It is disturbed muscular and glandular activity that is the way it appears to an external observer.

Components of Emotions

There are three components of emotions: 1. Cognition, 2. Feelings, and, 3. Behavior

Cognition

The cognition process starts by situation caused to motivate us in different emotional levels of anxiety and curiosity for evaluation.

Feelings

Feelings give rise to many physiological processes in the cardiovascular system and produce increased blood pressure and change in sexual urge. The strong feeling of disgust leads to face conflicts, frustrations, and even mental illness. These are stimulants in changes in functioning of nervous system and prompt electrochemical activities.

Behavior

Behavior is observable by facial expressions, by different postures or verbal or nonverbal communication. Nonverbal communication is more prominent in emotional behavior of human beings. Even in animals and birds also, they react according to the external and internal atmosphere of their surroundings.

The nonverbal communications are also common in human activities such as smile, facial feelings, eyebrow, folds in forehead in expression of disinterest, carelessness, fear, and anxiety. One of the most influential and important researchers in the field of emotion is Ekman. Here are a couple of examples from Ekman's work:

Changes During Emotions

Changes during emotions are divided into external and internal changes.

External Changes

There are many external or observable changes during emotion.

In some of the emotional situations, noticeable change appears in sound of aggression, breaking in speech, flow of saliva while speaking, etc. Experiments have proved that emotions can be identified on the basis of voice.

Facial expressions are easily noticeable by involvement of high level of emotional changes while breathing, sweating, crying, laughing, terror with shivering, etc. We can also identify emotion experienced by a person by looking at his face wrinkles on forehead, redness in eyes, and erection of hair on the skin.

Internal Changes

Internal change is very difficult to notice compared to external changes in emotions.

- **Galvanic Skin Response (GSR):** The physiological changes may be possible to measure by using Galvanic Skin Response. It helps in measuring of fluctuations in electrical conductivity of skin at the moment of high activity levels of sweat glands.
- **Polygraph:** "Lie detector" is used to measure the subtle variations in muscle tension, heart rate, etc. These are associated high or low levels of emotions involved in cognitive processes of thinking, memory, attention, etc.

The Physiological Response

The physiological responses are changes in physical symptoms during sickness like stomach pain, nausea, giddiness, stress, anxiety, fear, irregular levels in heartbeat, etc. Rapid breathing is controlled by the sympathetic nervous system.

The autonomic nervous system controls involuntary body responses such as blood flow and digestion.

The sympathetic nervous system controls our fearful emotions and is activated to face the challenges in fight-flight reaction. It is an internal change of emotions.

In body-mind relation, the brain function is to maintain emotional levels of individuals. The primary motives of hunger, thirst, and sleep are active in controlling the emotional behavior. These are also influences of internal changes in emotions by verbal and nonverbal communication.

After the emergency or emotional situation is over, the next step is to restore the energy spent during emotion. This work is carried on by parasympathetic division.

The emotional changes in human body are associated with central nervous system. The sympathetic and parasympathetic nervous system has major role in physical activities of body and mind functions. The function of endocrine glands has more influence on human behavior. Adrenaline gets circulated all over the body and stimulates vital organs leading to the following internal changes.

The emotional changes focus on rate of heartbeat, increase of blood levels, respiration, and increase of sugar levels in human body.

The appetite is low it affects the function of GI tract. It leads to dilation of pupils, low levels of secretion of saliva, and mouth will become dry.

Some experts believed that the social circumstances like culture, climate, terror, and war are basic universal emotions experienced by people in different areas of the world. Some are common emotions in feeling of happy, sad, anger, and anxiety. The mentally healthy person reacts to all these according to the situation. The abnormality is also noticed by failure of changes associated to human behavior.

Theories of Emotions

The James–Lange Theory of Emotion (Fig. 4.18)

In the 1880s, two theorists, psychologist **William James** and physiologist **Carl Lange,** independently proposed an idea that challenged common sense beliefs about emotion. This idea, which came to be known as the James-Lange theory, is that people experience emotion because they perceive their bodies' physiological responses to external events. According to this theory, an external stimulus leads to a physiological reaction. In this theory, our emotional reaction is after the bodily emotion.

For example: The person hears huge sounds and tries to close ears by physical activity. We notice these physiological changes and interpret them as our body's preparation for fearful situation. We experience fear.

We perceive the situation and will produce emotion. We will react to this situation. The same bodily changes occur in different kinds of emotional experiences. Our heart beat increases in both situations—happiness and unhappiness.

Cannon–Bard Theory of Emotion (Fig. 4.19)

The physiologist **Walter Cannon** disagreed with the James-Lange theory, posing three main arguments against it.

This theory states that we feel emotions and experience physiological reactions such as sweating, trembling, and muscle tension. Simultaneously, it is suggested that emotions result when the thalamus sends a message to the brain in response to a stimulus, resulting in a physiological reaction.

Cannon-Bard theory says that felt emotion and the bodily reactions in emotions are independent of each other, both are occurring simultaneously. James-Lange theory first responses physiologically to a stimulus, the cerebral cortex determines type of emotion experienced by the human being.

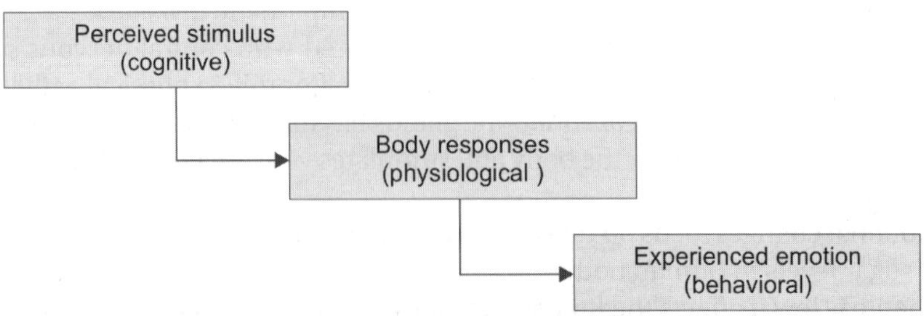

Fig. 4.18: James-Lange theory of emotion

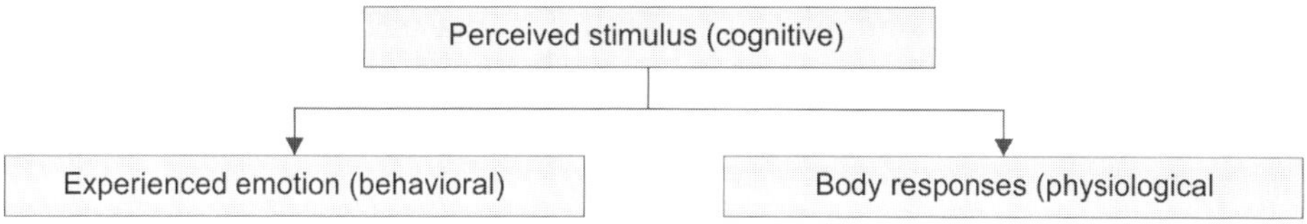

Fig. 4.19: Cannon Bard theory of emotion

Cannon–Bard expressed that impulses are sent simultaneously to cerebral cortex and peripheral nervous system. Thus, the response to the stimulus and the stimulus are experienced at the same time but independently.

For example, when someone is in a dark alley alone, a sudden sound usually provokes an immediate experience of fear, while the physical "symptoms" of fear generally follow that feeling. Neither one causes the other. The brain gets a message that causes the experience of emotion at the same time that the autonomic nervous system gets a message that causes physiological arousal.

Schachter-Singer Two-factor Theory of Emotion (Fig. 4.20)

In 1960s, **Stanley Schachter** and **Jerome Singer** proposed a different theory to explain emotion. They said that people's experience of emotion depends on two factors: physiological arousal and the cognitive interpretation of that arousal. When people perceive physiological symptoms of arousal, they look for an environmental explanation of this arousal. The label people give an emotion depends on what they find in their environment.

Schachter and Singer agree with the **James–Lange theory** that people infer emotions when they experience physiological arousal. But they also agree with the Cannon–Bard theory that the same pattern of physiological arousal can give rise to different emotions.

Schachter and Singer thought that the intensity of emotion depends upon cognitive appraisal of the situation. Thus, people experience internal arousal, become aware of the arousal, seek an explanation for it, identify an external cue, and finally label the cue.

Evolution Theories

More than a century ago, in the 1870s, **Charles Darwin** proposed that emotions evolved because they had adaptive value. In social interactions, it gives chances of feeling of love and affection in human bondage. It is gained from family, friends, neighbors, etc. Emotions motivate people to respond quickly to stimuli in the environment, which helps improve the chances of success and survival.

For example, fear evolved because it helped people to act in ways that enhanced their chances of survival. Recent evolutionary theories of emotion also consider emotions to be

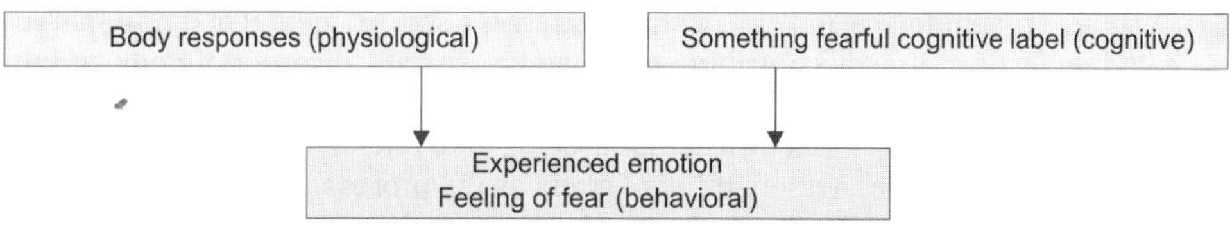

Fig. 4.20: Schachter-Singer two-factor theory of emotion

innate responses to stimuli. Evolutionary theorists believe that all human cultures share several primary emotions, including happiness, contempt, surprise, disgust, anger, fear, and sadness. Understanding the emotions of other people and animals also plays a crucial role in safety and survival.

Emotion Influence on Health

Emotional irregularities are causes for both physical and mental ill health in human beings. The increase of emotions causes to stomach pain, headache, ulcers, back pain, chest pain, constipation, etc. These are also caused by distress.

By Department of Cardiology, KIMS—Secunderabad Branch (KIMS, one of the top heart hospitals in Hyderabad, has a long history of pioneering coronary artery disease treatment).
(Dr B Bhaskar Rao (Fig 4.21) - Managing Director and Chief Executive Officer of KIMS)

Many risk factors for coronary artery disease (CAD) are:
- High blood cholesterol and triglyceride levels (a type of fat found in the blood)
- High blood pressure
- Diabetes and prediabetes
- Overweight and obesity
- Smoking
- Lack of physical activity
- Unhealthy diet
- Stress

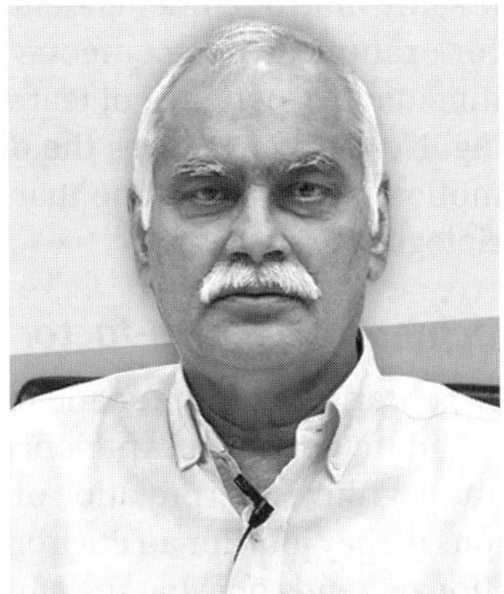

Fig. 4.21: Dr B Bhaskar Rao, Times Healthcare Achievers Award 2017- Life-time achiever of the year in Cardiology and Cardiothoracic surgery

Following a healthy lifestyle can help us to prevent or control many CHD (cardiac heart diseases) risk factors.

Because many lifestyle habits begin during childhood, parents and families should encourage their children to make heart-healthy choices. This may prevent CHD from worsening. Even if you are in your seventies or eighties, a healthy lifestyle can lower your risk of dying from CHD.

Poor emotional health affects our body. It makes us weak in facing infections. The increase of feelings of stress leads to negligence of healthcare in individuals. It creates disinterest in functional activities of body such as physical exercises, intake of food, and medicines for well-being of the individual. It is the major cause for decreased life span of people in society. Its extremes lead to mental disorders or even suicides.

STRESS AND STRESSOR

Stress: A state of psychological tension or strain. Stress is a state of mental or emotional strain. Stress can directly or indirectly contribute to general or specific disorder of body and mind. Stress is difficult to define because researchers approach it in different ways. Some use the term *stress* to refer to circumstances that threaten well-being or to refer to the response people have to threatening circumstances. Others think of stress as the process of evaluating and coping with threatening circumstances.

Stress is not always harmful. The low levels of stress can help for better performance. The body reacts to stressors by initiating a complete sequence of response.

Hans Selye (1945) developed stress theory—"It is not stress that kills us. It is our reaction to it."

Types of Stress

- **Eustress—good stress**—positive stress
  It is helpful and assists the drive toward achievement and success.
- **Distress—bad stress—negative stress (Fig. 4.22)**
  Chronic stress leads to physiological disorders. It affects life in adverse manner and it is common cause of ill-health in our society.

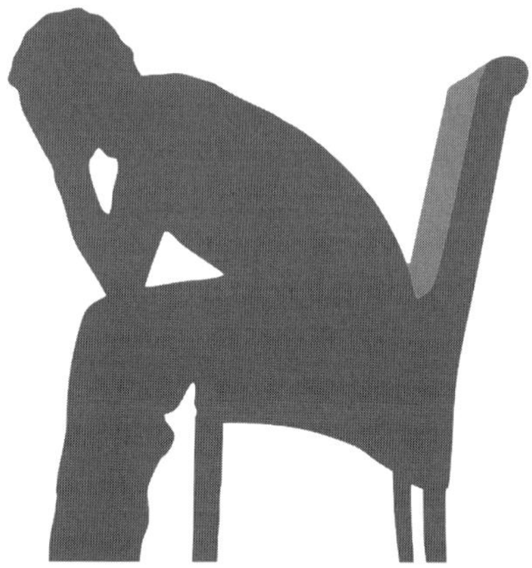

Fig. 4.22: Condition of negative stress

Physical Stress

- Poor appetite or over eating
- Feeling tired and fatigue
- Various aches and pain—headache, body ache, and muscle pain
- Nausea and abdominal pain, increased nail-biting, migraine, obesity
- Sleep problems
- Falling sick very often—fever, cough, and diarrhea.

Mental Stress

- Nervousness and anxiety
- Moodiness, irritation, inability to relax
- Excessive anger or depression
- Being easily upset
- Poor self-confidence
- Lack of concentration
- Poor performance in studies.

Stressors are psychologically or physically demanding events or circumstances. Stressors include either positive or negative life events. Research links stressors to increased susceptibility to physical illnesses such as heart disease as well as to psychological problems such as anxiety and depression.

Mallet and Whaley defined stressor—In technical sense, however, it refers to "a type of stimulus that occurs in sufficient amount to cause stress".

Catastrophic Events

Large earthquakes, hurricanes, wars.

Major life changes—positive or negative: Marriage, divorce, death of a parent, beginning a new job, starting college.

Distress leads to alcoholism, drug abuse, interpersonal relation difficulties, depression, anxiety, and even suicide.

Minor hassles: Standing in line, traffic jams, noisy environments.

A stressful event can trigger the "fight-or-flight" response as adrenaline and cortisol to surge through the body.

Coping with Stress

Coping may have described as dealing with change for success. It is searching for solution to focused problems connected to stress. Coping mechanisms can help in reduction of distress.

Coping

According to Folkman and Lazrus (1991), Coping is defined as "the cognitive and behavioral efforts to manage specific external and or internal demands that are appraised as taxing to a changing environment or specific problem or situation".

LEARN to manage stress

- L—Laugh—watching comedy shows, reading jokes
- E—Extracurricular activities—games, sports, aerobics
- A—Avoid negative thoughts
- R—Relaxation techniques—PMR (progressive muscular relaxation) technique, Yoga, meditation, dancing, listening music, watching TV
- N—Normal life

During stress, some people consume excessive amount of alcohol and smoke excessively. A high fat diet contributes to many forms of cancers as well as cardiovascular diseases. People who engage a healthy lifestyle—good diet, good sleep, rest, and body exercises—can balance stress levels. It helps to expand life span.

Tips to Reduce Stress

- Time management
- Drink 8 or 10 glasses of water every day
- Prefer to eat Vitamin C-rich food
- Eat nutritious food **(Fig. 4.23)**
- Move body frequently
- Do not sit for more than one hour
- Reduce your intake of alcohol
- Make face to face connection with the people of priority
- Do something to enjoy a day—good conversation, gardening, enjoy with pet dogs or animals, swimming, dancing, playing music instrument and listening music, watching TV (comedy shows), plan a picnic, window shopping.

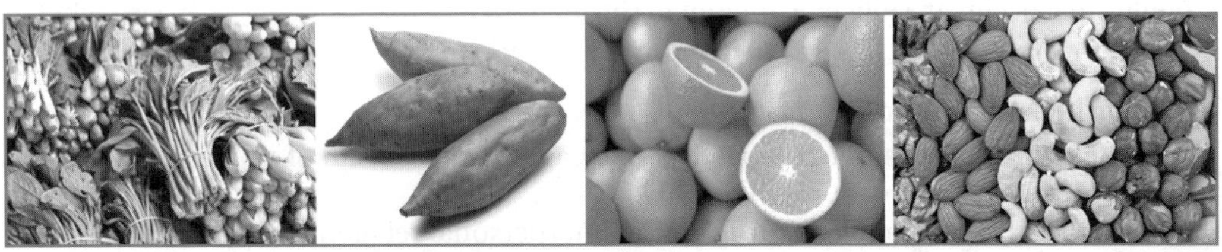

Fig. 4.23: Healthy diet to manage stress (dark green vegetables, sweet potato, oranges and nuts)

Coping strategies can be either positive or negative. Positive or adaptive strategies decrease the amount of stress perceived and experienced. Adaptive coping helps the person to deal effectively with stressful events and minimize distress associated with them. The effectiveness of individual's coping is influenced by a number of factors like intensity of the stressors and past experience. The experience of positive emotions functions to assist high-resilient individuals in their ability to recover effectively from daily stress.

ATTITUDE

Attitude is a psychological construct. It is a mental and emotional entity that inheres in or characterizes a person. An attitude is a predisposition to react in a persistent and characteristic manner of situation. It is precipitated through a responsive expression toward a person, place, thing, or event which turns and influences the individual's thought and action.

In 1874, three ladies applied for admission to the Madras Medical College. The college officials were in favor of having lady doctors in the country, but were concerned about their training phase.

An attitude toward coeducation changed in modern societies. Long back there was lack of literacy in females in Indian society. Most of the girls were encouraged to get education by availability of schools and colleges in their localities. Most of the girls were satisfied to be as house wife after marriage. In modern days, education for girls is encouraged and they are working in different organizations based on their skills.

The behavioral implications of social attitudes and their consequences in society can, thus, be far-reaching. It is for this reason that attitudes are among the central concepts of social psychology.

Attitudes accompanied by strong feelings are called sentiments. Social psychologists have given more definitions on this concept. It is like belief or opinion that includes an evaluation of some object, person, or even along a continuum from negative to positive.

Kimball Young defined "an attitude is predisposition to respond, in a persistent and characteristic manner, in reference to some situation, idea, value, material, object, person, (or) group of persons.

Young K defined attitude as "a learned and more or less generalized and an effective tendency or predisposition to respond in a rather persistent and characteristic manner, usually positively or negatively (for or against in reference to some situation, idea, value, material object, or class) of such objects or person or group of persons".

Gordon W Alport defined "An attitude to be a mental and neural state of readiness, organized through experience, exerting a directive or dynamic influence upon the individual's response to all objects and situations with which it is related".

Generally, aptitude is categorized by evaluation, target, and pre-disposition. Evaluation involves likes and dislikes. The person chooses goal by his interest toward particular point. It shows the attitude of the person on specific areas in both personal and professional life of an individual. Predisposition is an approach to some objects, people, and events to avoid others because of corresponding positive or negative attitudes.

Attitude Change-Approach

The facts determined on attitudes are environment, education, and experience. Social agencies like family, school, neighborhood, state, and religion are more influenced changes in attitudes and goal setting.

Attitudes are acquired by thoughts, processes, and norms. Heredity is also influenced like environment in determinants of attitudes. The head of a traditional family, the village head, the religious priest, the social worker, the gang leader, the propagandist, etc., are all examples of people who influence the attitudes of others. With altruistic or selfish interests in mind, these people employ ways and means that are more intuitive than scientific. Numerous studies have been done on the subject matter of attitude change and over a dozen theories have been advanced to interpret and accommodate the facts related to the dynamics of attitude change.

The individual might also reject the new information and maintain the old cognitive structures. Another approach to attitude change may arise from an analysis of the functions which a particular attitude fulfills for a person. Attitude changes from direct experience.

PSYCHOMETRIC ASSESSMENT OF EMOTIONS AND ATTITUDES

Psychometric assessment of emotions**:** Emotions can be studied in the laboratory by conducting different experiments. It is important to judge the emotions.

The judgment of attitude is very difficult. Individuals are not strong to stick on a particular point or particular procedure. It makes difficult to assess attitudes. The psychometric assessments are done by conducting experiments. It is also difficult to get accurate results in assessing.

The individual has to select the appropriate emotion from the list and compare that emotion with photos and judge. In other experiments, a part of face is shown to a person and then he is asked to judge the emotions. Even by listening to only voice, not looking at the facial expressions, the emotions of a person can be judged. This can be demonstrated through experiments in laboratories.

Psychologists have developed many techniques to measure attitudes. The measurement technique depends upon the purpose. As stated above, our evaluations are expressed by terms such as liking-disliking, pro-anti, favoring-not favoring, positive-negative, etc. Most commonly used technique is self-report method.

Self-reporting may be in the form of expressing preferences to an interviewer or to write evaluations of something on a long questionnaire. The questionnaire must be in objective manner by model of like, dislike, good, bad, satisfactory, etc.

Public opinion (attitudes) polling is a self-reporting method, which includes survey, distributing pamphlets, and sending SMS on different topics, to know public trend in decision-making. It is more helpful in implementing of new programs in modern society.

Attitude scales: An attitude scale attempts to obtain a precise measure of the extremity of people's attitudes. The accuracy of the measurement can be increased by using many items that are all related to the same issue.

There are many attitude scales to measure attitudes.

- Thurston's equal appearing interval scale
- Likert's Summated rating scale
- Bogardus social distance scale.

In addition to the above methods, there are some involuntary behavioral measures which are used to measure the attitude indicators which are not under the voluntary control of the respondent.

For example, physiological measures such as Galvanic Skin Response (GSR), Electromyography (EMG), etc. These tests are not commonly used. Change of attitude can be experimentally shown by providing some information about an unknown person. In this experiment, a photo of a person will be shown along with some positive information.

After a gap of time, negative information about the same person will be presented. Then we can find out the effect of this new information on the change of attitude.

ALTERATIONS IN EMOTIONS

Some of the alterations in emotions are: Abrupt changes in mood, experiencing conflicting emotions at the same time about the same thing, displaying inappropriate emotional responses such as mania or euphoria (that is excessive joy), depression, and extreme sadness or despair.

CONCLUSION

In nursing profession, the knowledge of components of motivation helps in understanding patient's desires toward achievement of goal and causes of conflicts and frustration in social adjustment. Understanding and detailed study on secondary motives, observation on patient's priority in goal setting, and causes of inefficiency in achievement help the nurse in diagnosis and speedy recovery of illness. The theories of motivation guide the nurse in reduction of harmful desires and helps to healthy living of the patient.

The detailed study on emotion, changes, and altering techniques to controlling helps the nurse to motivate the patient in controlling severe health problems.

The stress management to organizing techniques and tips to reduce distress help the nurse to manage both her personal and professional life.

QUESTIONS

Essay Questions

1. Give an account of biological, social, and personal motives with reference to Maslow.
2. Explain types and theories of motivation and narrate conflict resolution.
3. A. Define emotion. B. Explain the theories of emotions. C. Narrate emotions in health and sickness.
4. A. Evaluate general theories of attitude. B. Explain factors involved in attitude change. C. Write in detail about psychometric assessment of attitude. D. Emotions. How emotions could be driving force for human behavior?
5. Define stress. List the stressors and explain adaptation and coping.

Short Answers

1. Conflict and frustration.
2. Illustrate the factors affecting behavior and attitudes.
3. Factors affecting attitude.
4. Write the nature and development of attitude.
5. Define conflict and explain conflict resolution.
6. Definition and types of motivation.
7. Explain source of stress.
8. Types of conflict and methods to solve it.
9. Explain types of attitudes.
10. Define conflict and frustration.

11. Mention any two features of variability in attitude.
12. List the salient features of motives and behavior.
13. Define the stress and discuss about adoption and coping.
14. Evaluate the theories of emotions.
15. Enlist the sources of stressors.
16. Define attitude change.
17. Write the meaning of social motives.
18. Physiological changes during emotions.
19. Stress and coping styles.
20. Emotional adjustment and illness.
21. Explain the behavior of attitude.

Brief Questions

1. Define frustration.
2. Enlist the sources of stressors.
3. Social motives.
4. Mention the components of emotions.
5. Stress and coping.
6. Mention any two effects of stressors.
7. Differentiate between emotions and feelings.
8. Define biological motive.
9. Differentiate between aptitude and attitude.
10. Enlist the types of attitudes.
11. Write the differences between eustress and distress.
12. Conflicts.
13. Enumerate the types of conflicts.

Fill in the Blanks

1. Motivation is the study of goal-directed ________. (behavior).
2. The four ________ of motivation are need, drive, response, and goal. (components)
3. McClelland's theory of motivation explains achievement, ________, and power. (affiliation)
4. Abraham H Maslow developed the hierarchy of needs consisting of physiological, safety and security, self-esteem, psychological happiness, and ________. (self-actualization)
5. Four types of conflicts are approach-approach conflict, ________, avoidance-avoidance conflict, and multiple-approach conflict. (approach-avoidance conflict)
6. Emotion is derived from the Latin word ________. (emovere)
7. Love, pleasure, and affection are ________ emotions. (positive)
8. Polygraph is ________ used to measure the subtle variations in muscle tension, heart rate, etc. (lie detector)
9. Stress is a state of psychological ________ or strain. (tension)
10. Eustress is positive stress and ________ is negative stress. (distress)
11. Attitudes accompanied by strong feelings are called ________. (sentiments)
12. Thurston's Equal Appearing Interval Scale is used to measure ________. (attitude).

Multiple Choice Questions

1. Components of motives ....
   a. Goal
   b. Need
   c. Both
2. McClelland's motivational theory based on ....
   a. Affiliation
   b. Power
   c. Both
3. Avoidance and avoidance conflict occurs in between two ....
   a. Positive
   b. Negative
   c. Positive and negative
4. Approach and approach conflict is a conflict between two .... goals.
   a. Positive
   b. Negative
   c. Positive and negative
5. Motion is derived from the ....
   a. Movere
   b. Emovere
   c. None
6. GSR means ....
   a. Galvanic skin response
   b. Motivational response
   c. Galvanic skin regulation

Answers

1. c	2. c	3. b	4. a	5. b	6. a

5 CHAPTER

Personality

Learning Objectives

- Personality
- Definitions, topography, types, theories
- Psychometric assessment of personality
- Alterations in personality
- Applications

Personality is the total quality of an individual's behavior as it is shown in thinking, attitudes, interests, and mannerism associated in social relations of human life.

Every person is different from each other in skin color, features, height, weight, etc. The siblings are not same in the same family. In one family, each child may be different in habits, attitudes, and physical traits. Some people may be intelligent and some may be dull in understanding, learning, and perceiving. It depends on their physical and mental abilities.

Personality studies the variations among individuals. Personality expresses the psychological processes of human beings in day-to-day life. The psychology studied on personality is called personality psychology. Many personality development programs are developed in modern society to improve the healthy development in both personal and social life of the people. These programs help the individual and group to motivate to be mentally healthy and to lead comfortable life by facing challenges like success and failure in their daily activities. It helps in modification of human behavior. These developmental programs encourage person to manage good mental health by employment, administration, business, and family life to face distress, anxiety, and depressed tendencies. Many approaches have been taken in studying personality, including biological, cognitive, learning, and trait-based theories, as well as psychodynamic and humanistic approaches.

The trait-based approach has yielded multiple conceptions of personality, including a number of five-factor models, Eysenck's traits, and Cloninger's temperament and character traits.

Personality is dynamic. Personality characteristics influence the person and motivate by cognition processes of learning and attention.

Personality has been derived from the Latin word **"persona"** which means "mask" used by the actors to change their appearance. One cannot determine it exactly because it varies from culture to culture and time to time.

For example: The king in the battle fights to protect the country and people, in another way he is a criminal by killing others in war. A killer is considered criminal in peace time and hero in war. Personality also refers to the feelings, social adjustments, and behavior consistently exhibited over time that strongly influences one's expectations, self-perceptions, values, and attitudes.

Another example, teacher punishes children for mischievous activities of students in class as his duty, another way he has to manage patience in dealing matters in life with children.

Personality is the quality or state of being a person.

DEFINITIONS

Watson: "Personality is the sum of activities that can be discovered by actual observations over a long enough period of time to give reliable information."

Gordon Alport (1937): "Personality is the dynamic within the individual of those psychosexual systems that determine his unique adjustment to his environment."

NL Munn: Personality may be defined as the most characteristic integration of an individual structure, modes of behavior, interests, attitudes, capacities, abilities, and aptitudes.

Mc. Diugall JW: "Personality is a synthetic unity of mental features and functions in their interplay."

American Psychiatric Association-1987: "Personality refers to deeply ingrained patterns of behavior, which include the way one relates to perceive and think about environment and one's self."

The personality dimensions **(Fig. 5.1)** help in understanding the theories. The major theories include dispositional (trait) perspective, psychodynamic, humanistic, biological, behavioral, evolutionary, and social learning perspectives.

In psychological education and training, the study of the nature of personality and its psychological development is usually reviewed as a prerequisite course in abnormal psychology and clinical psychology.

THE TYPE APPROACH (FIG. 5.2)

The type approach explains human personality and behavior based on structure, physiological, blood type, and secretion.

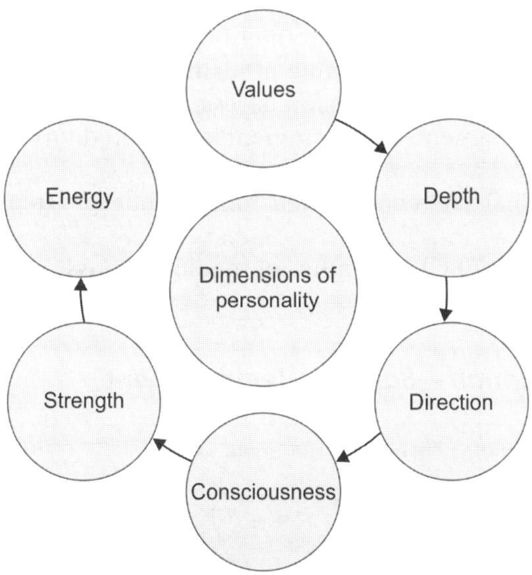

Fig. 5.1: The personality dimensions

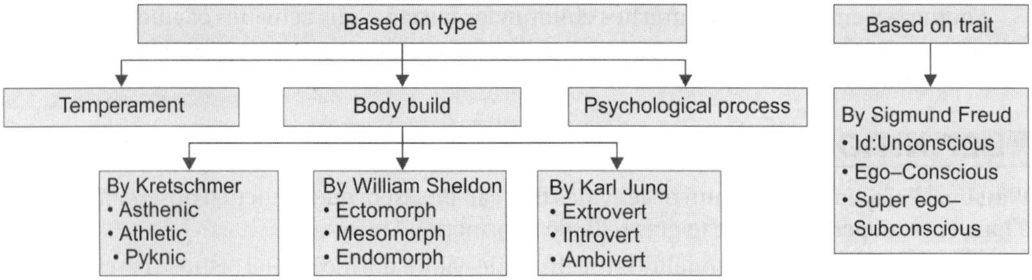

Fig. 5.2: A type approach

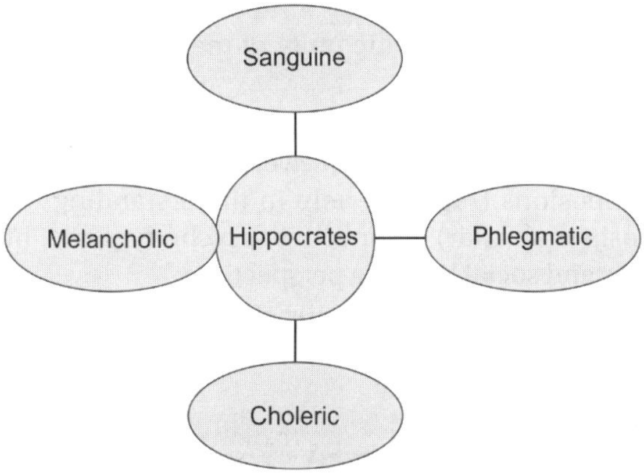

Fig. 5.3: Hippocrates classification of personality—based on temperament

Personality Based on Temperament

Individual's personality based on temperament confuses in decision-making by quality of judgment. Personality is more valuable in justification on several issues. Sometimes the person reacts by irritation, depression, stress, and other changes to get aggression, anxiety, and other temperaments. Temperament is the hereditary and emotional aspect of personality.

The theory of individual differences started from the concept of temperament suggested by Hippocrates and Galen.

Hippocrates (about 400 BC), the father of medicine, classified people into four types **(Fig. 5.3)** as per temperament.

Hippocrates Classification—Based on Temperament

- Phlegmatic—Calm, slow-moving, unexcitable, unemotional
- Melancholic—Depressed, pessimistic
- Sanguin—Cheerful, confident, optimistic
- Choleric—Irritable, hot tempered (yellow bile)

Type Based on Body Build (Physiological Type)

- Kretschmer
- William Sheldon

Kretschmer (1925) Classification

Kretschmer divided people into three types based on body structure.

Kretschmer (1925) classification
1. Asthenic—Introvert, tall, thin, sensitive (unsociable, shy, pessimist, alone)
2. Athletic—Active, aggressive, well-developed muscular body (energetic, optimistic, good in adjustment)
3. Pyknic—Extrovert, round, and fat. (social and helping nature)

William Sheldon

William Sheldon (1954) divided **(Fig. 5.4)** people into three types **(Fig 5.2)** according to body build and behavior.

William Sheldon
1. Endomorph—Plumb, soft, fat, and round—sociable even tempered and relaxed
2. Mesomorph—Heavy set and muscular—Physically active and noisy
3. Ectomorph—Tall, thin, and flat chested, self-conscious—shy and reserved.

Based on Psychological Process (Emotion, Stress)

Dr Karl Jung classification—based on sociability

Extroverts—Sociable, friendly not easily upset by difficulties, politician's social workers, lawyers, and salesmen.
The extroverts are service-oriented and manage good social relation.

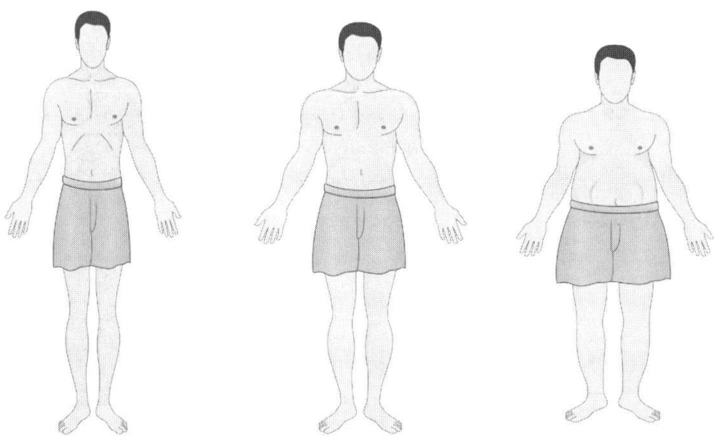

Fig. 5.4: Sheldon's classification of personality by body build and behavior

Introverts: Shy, reserved, isolated, easily embarrassed—Philosophers, scientists, and writers. Planned life, deep thinking, less social interactions, and prefer to be alone.

Ambiverts: There are very few people who are pure extroverts or introverts. Majority of people are ambiverts having qualities of extroverts and introverts in different proportions.

Type A and Type B Personality Theory

During 1950, Meyer Friedman and his co-workers defined what they called Type A and Type B behavior patterns **(Fig. 5.5)**.

TRAIT THEORIES OF PERSONALITY

In trait approach, the personality depends on traits of honesty, shy, lazy, dull, etc. These are constant patterns of behavior interpreted in different situations.

Play for fun and relaxation, instead of exhibiting their superiority without the feeling of inferiority.

The Major Trait Theories of Personality

The trait theories of personality are based on psychodynamics. It is influenced by biological process of human behavior, social learning, and evolutional process. The nature of personality is psychological development applied in fields of abnormal and clinical psychology.

Psychoanalytic Theory

Psychoanalytic theory explains human behavior in terms of the interaction of various components of personality. Behavior is divided into individual interactions and develops in human behavior.

Freud's Psychoanalytic Theory

Sigmund Freud (6 May 1856–23 September 1939) **(Fig. 5.6)** gave one of the most famous psychoanalytic theory which formed the basis for many current psychodynamic theories.

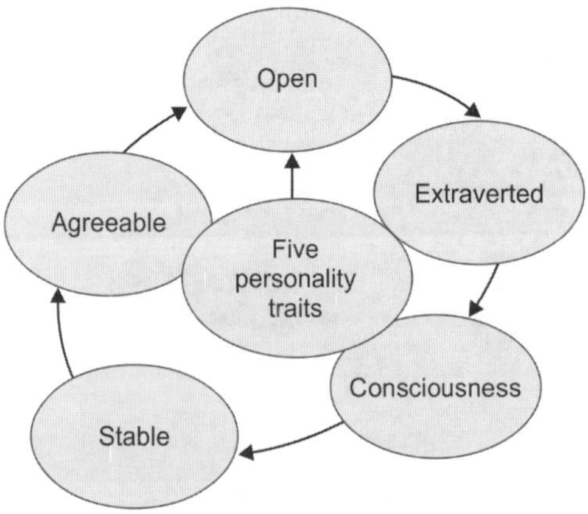

Fig. 5.5: Personality traits

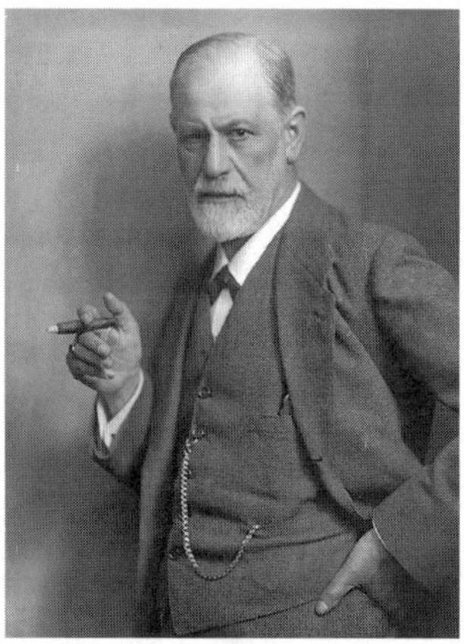

Fig. 5.6: Sigmund Freud

It is more popular in modern psychology. Freud's theory placed prominence on dynamic, unconscious psychological conflicts.

Sigmund Freud's theory of personality stresses the influences of unconscious fears, desires, and motivation on thoughts and behavior. Freud theory of personality development reveals the willingness or interest aspects in interpretation. Freud focused on internal growth of personality. It is called as psychodynamics.

Structure of Personality

Freud classified structure into three elements of Id, ego, and super-ego **(Fig. 5.7)**.

Id	Ego	Superego
Instincts	Reality	Morality
(I wanted to do that now)	(May be we can compromise)	(It is not right to do that)

The Id: The id is composed of biological components of drives and aggression. It is self-centered. It stands on "pleasure principle" for self-satisfaction. The id needs immediate satisfaction. In this way, the id resolves tension and anxiety. It is the development of the ego and the super ego that allows people to control the basic instincts.
For example: I need to eat right this second.

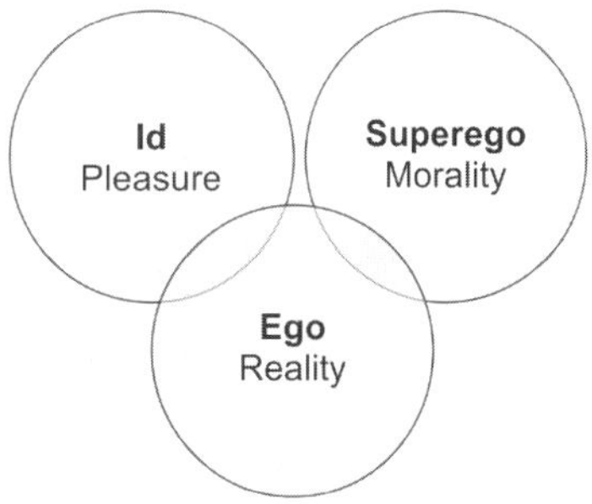

Fig. 5.7: Freud's structural elements of personality

The Ego: The ego is judging principle between id and super ego. The ego operates in our preconscious and conscious mind. It stands on reality principle in conscious level. Freud used the word ego to mean a sense of self, but later revised it to mean a set of psychic functions such as judgment, tolerance, reality testing, control, planning, and defending. The ego must mediate the demands of the id, the superego, and reality.

Superego: Each stage is processed through Freud's concept of the human mind as a three tier system consisting of the superego, the ego, and the id. The superego functions at both preconscious and conscious levels. It is developed through the cultural environment and learning from social contacts such as parents and other elder members of family. It focuses on judgment and analyzation on thoughts of ego. The person feels guilty by opposing the thoughts of superego. It is like a screen test on behavior.

Freud believed that the id, ego, and super ego were in constant conflict with one another; the ego controls the demands of the id and the superego supervises the behavior of the ego.

For example: You cannot do that because you are in the middle of an important meeting (superego).

Personality Dynamics (Structure of the Mind and Body)

Freud divided personality into three interacting structures. He assumed that the thoughts are determined by internal psychological thoughts and feelings.

Topographical Description

Freud described the levels of unconsciousness, consciousness, and subconsciousness **(Fig. 5.8)**.

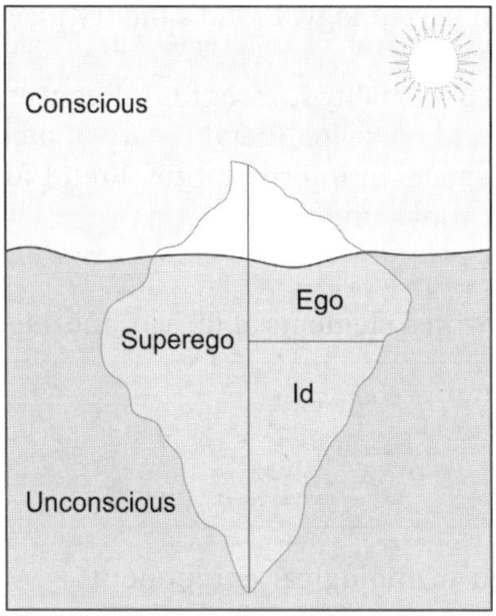

Fig. 5.8: Levels of consciousness

The unconscious—Id: The mind is not given attention toward right or wrong by performance. It needs pleasure in achievement. It includes desires, fears, and phobias. It consists of biological impulses or drives like food and drink to avoid pain and to gain pleasure.

The conscious—ego: The mind functions on awareness of present thoughts, feelings, and sensations. It stands on reality and motivates an individual to behave in a rational way. The main difference between id and ego is the subjective reality of the mind in ego. The id cannot directly satisfy itself by obtaining needs from environment.

The preconscious or subconscious–superego: The mind and body interact with each other. It motivates moral process of thoughts and feelings in mind. The level of preconscious prevents certain unacceptable memories, disturbed unconscious memories reaching to the conscious mind. The preconscious can prevent from emotional thoughts which are cause for mental illness.

According to Freud's structural model, the personality is divided into the id, ego, and super ego.

Freud's theory places central importance on dynamic, unconscious psychological conflicts.

Psychosexual Stages

Freud focused on individual psychosexual development. According to Freud, the child develops through unresolved conflicts between physiological drives and social environment. These are determined from their childhood experiences. These are helpful in determination of future developmental changes of an individual. It also helps in modification of human behavior in their adulthood.

Freud's theory of the psychosexual stages **(Fig. 5.9)** comprises mainly of—oral, anal, phallic, and genital—the theory postulates that problems move from one stage to another in adult personality. It rises in personal and social environment in modification of behavior. Hence, there are adult personality traits that arise from childhood experiences. Further opposite patterns can be seen as reactions to the same problem.

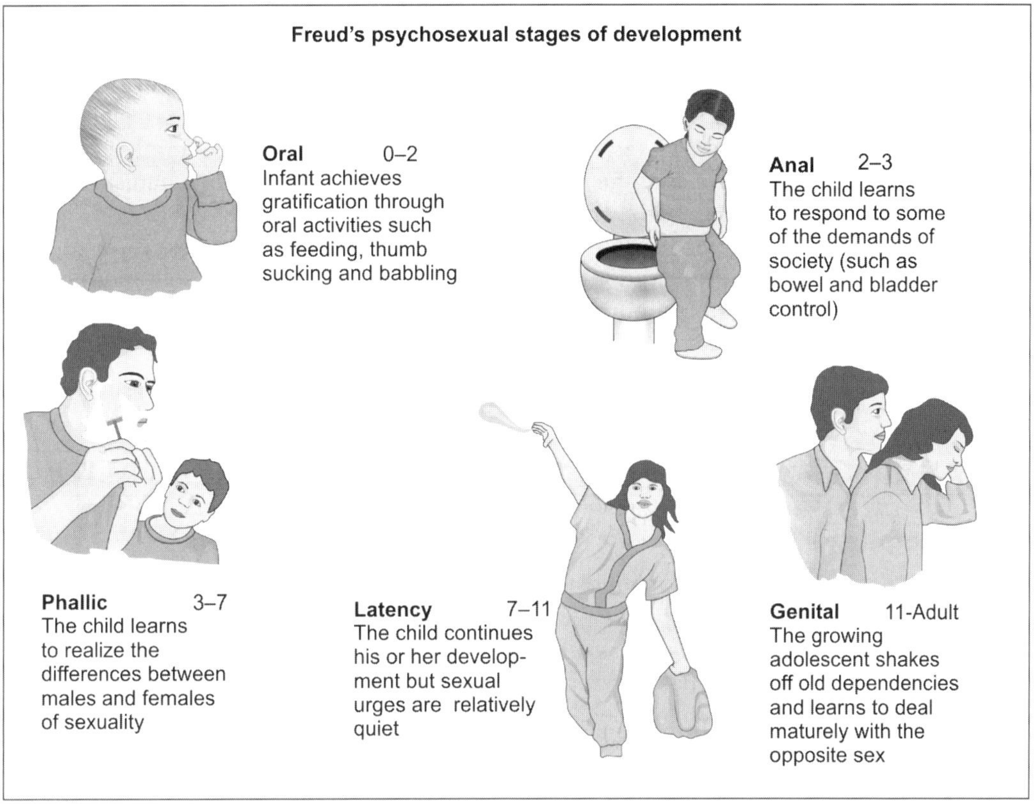

Fig. 5.9: Freud's theory on psychosexual development
(*Source:* By Allyn and Bacon)

The oral stage (birth to 1.5 years): The oral stage is from birth to one and half year. Pleasure is obtained through stimulation of the mouth as in nursing or thumb sucking. The goal of this stage is to guide in proper way of sucking, eating, biting, talking, etc. Some children are very active in intake of food, digestion, grasping and managing power in their behavior. In modern days, most of children are influenced by mobiles by imitation from parents in early months of life.

Thus, both oral optimists and pessimists live with their problems over early feeding but in very different ways.

The anal stage (1.5 to 3 years): The Freudians believe this phase is associated with later hostile, sadistic, and obsessive behavior. Sometimes the children may learn by punishment in toilet training.

The phallic stage (3 to 7 years): The phallic stage provides pleasure in healthy development to sexual attraction.

The girl develops affection for their father. The 5-year-old boy supposedly (and unconsciously) feels love toward mother and not shows interest to his father. Pride and doubt, boldness, and timidity are personality characteristics associated with the phallic stage.

Latency (7 to 11 years): The latency stage is a center of major pleasure and dominant feelings of love and attention to opposite sex by this puberty stage. It is necessary in maturation of adult personality to develop before puberty. The child continues his or her development; sexual urges are relatively quiet in this stage.

Genital stage (11 to 18 years): The growing adolescent learns to deal maturity with the opposite sex. The experience of previous stages allows mind to develop health sexual feelings and behavior. The individual turns to analyze healthy social relationships employment and enjoyment of life. Freud stated that the individual tries to imply defense mechanisms to face the complicated situation from social environment.

The channeling and release of sexual (libido) and aggressive energies, which ensues from the "Eros" (sex; instinctual self-preservation) and "Thanatos" (death; instinctual self-annihilation) drives, respectively, are major components of his theory.

One of Sigmund Freud's earlier associates, Alfred Adler, agreed with Freud that early childhood experiences are important to development and believed birth order may influence personality development.

LEARNING AND BEHAVIORIST THEORIES OF PERSONALITY

Social Cognitive Theories

In cognitive theory, behavior is explained as guided by cognitions (e.g., expectations) about the world, especially those about other people. Cognitive theories are theories of personality that emphasize cognitive processes, such as thinking and judging.

Behaviorists explain personality in terms of the effects external stimuli have on behavior. The approaches used to analyze the behavioral aspect of personality are known as behavioral theories or learning-conditioning theories. These approaches were a radical shift away from Freudian philosophy. One of the major tenets of this concentration of personality psychology is a strong emphasis on scientific thinking and experimentation.

The behavioral theorist BF Skinner shared that mutual interaction of the person or organism and not a victim of his environment. The behavioral approach reinforces attention in obtaining goals. The child cries to get attention of their mother in responding to the consequences.

According to operant conditioning or instrumental conditioning theories, people's behavior is formed by processes of promoting stimulus responses.

Ivan Pavlov, popularly known in conditioned reflexes of classical conditioning, involved dogs which led him to discover the foundation of behaviorism.

Albert Bandura, a social learning theorist, suggested that the forces of memory and emotions are influenced by force of environment.

Bandura was known mostly for his "Bobo doll experiment" **(Fig. 5.10)**. During these experiments, Bandura video-taped a college student kicking and verbally abusing a bobo doll. He then showed this video to a class of kindergarten children who were getting ready to go out to play. When they entered the play room, they saw bobo dolls and some hammers.

People observed these children at play and saw a group of children beating the doll. Bandura stated that human behaviour influenced by observational learning. Since 1970, this type of guidance has been more applicable in setting goals of education and counseling field.

Walter Mischel (1999) has also defended a cognitive approach to personality. His work refers to "Cognitive Affective Units," and considers factors such as encoding of stimuli, goal-setting, and self-regulatory beliefs.

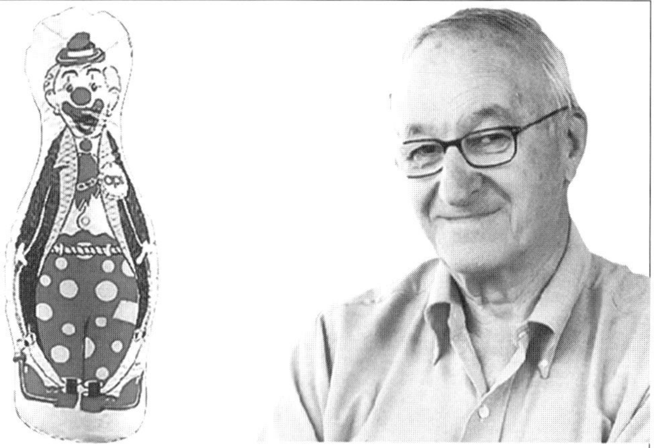

A Bobo Doll Albert Bandura

Fig. 5.10: Bobo doll experiment—Albert Bandura

Cognitive experiential theory (CET) is another cognitive personality theory. Developed by Seymour Epstein, CET stated that humans are operated by inter-dependence of both experimental and rational systems. But both determine our goals, thoughts, and behavior. It is fast and emotion-driven. The rational system is slow and logic-driven. These two systems interact to determine our goals, thoughts, and behavior.

Humanistic theories of personality: The personality development focuses upon the development of self which is called humanism.

Humanistic psychology focuses on subjective experiences of persons as opposed to forced, definitive factors that determine behavior.

Rogers and Maslow were among a group of psychologists that worked together for a decade to produce the Journal of Humanistic Psychology. This journal was primarily focused on viewing individuals as a whole, rather than focusing solely on separate traits and processes within the individual. The theorists, Carl Roger and Abraham Maslow, rejected the internal conflicts of Freud's view of mechanistic nature of behaviorism.

Maslow spent much of his time studying on self-actualization. They believe that every individual is creative and responsible in choosing to fulfill their desires or self-actualization. Maslow believes all who are interested in growth move toward self-actualizing (growth, happiness, satisfaction) views. Many of these people demonstrate a trend in dimensions of their personalities.

Humanistic therapy typically relies on the client for information of the past and its effect on the present; therefore, the client dictates the type of guidance the therapist may initiate. This allows for an individualized approach to therapy.

Five-factor Model or the Five Trait Theory of Personality

The five-factor model theory organizes personality traits under five categories.

The key five traits **(Fig. 5.11)** of human personality are similar to the "Big Five" that Goldberg researched in 1993.

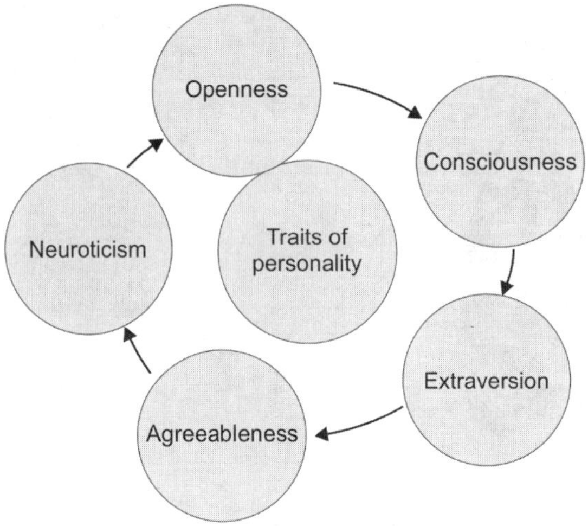

Fig. 5.11: Five-factor trait theory of personality

The traits are stable tendencies to behave in certain ways. It is not applicable in all situations of human life.

Personality traits are both changeable and stable. Most of the experts are accepting that changes appear more below the age of 30 years. The youth and adults are willing to show interest toward newness in changing attitudes.

The genetic features have a considerable influence on personality traits behavior.

Traits are useful in description of people and certain personality differences in behavior.

Evolutionary Theory

The word evolution means gradual development.

Charles Darwin is the founder of the Theory of Evolution of the species. The evolutionary approach to personality psychology is based on this theory.

Darwin Theory

"The possibility of linking humans with earlier apes by descent became clear only after 1859 with the publication of Charles Darwin **(Fig. 5.12)** on the Origin of Species, in which he argued for the idea of the evolution of new species from earlier ones."

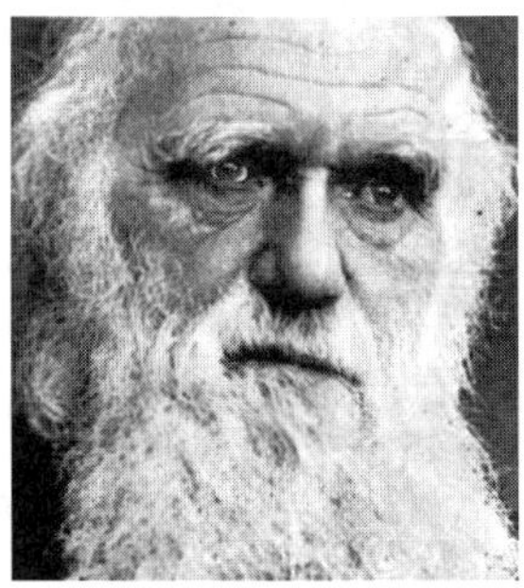

Fig. 5.12: Charles Darwin

This theory helps in understanding of individual differences based on personality and evolution. The organism adopts the changes to exist for survival and reproduction.

The theory of evolution has wide ranging implications on personality psychology. Personality viewed through the lens of evolutionary psychology places a great deal of emphasis on specific traits that are most likely to aid in survival and reproduction, such as conscientiousness, sociability, emotional stability, and dominance. Specific character traits develop and are selected for because they play an important and complex role in the social hierarchy of organisms. Such characteristics of this social hierarchy include the sharing of important resources, family and mating interactions, and the harm or help organisms can bestow upon one another.

PSYCHOMETRIC ASSESSMENT OF PERSONALITY

Personality can be determined through a variety of tests:
- Big Five Inventory (BFI)
- Minnesota Multiphasic Personality Inventory (MMPI)
- Rorschach Ink-blot Test
- Neurotic Personality Questionnaire or Eysenck's Personality questionnaire (EPQ).

Personality Tests

There are two major types of personality tests, projective and objective.

Projective tests assumed in an unconscious level and assess on stimulation of responses. These have been popular for the past 60 years in assessing personality.

Objective tests: Objective tests are based on conscious level and by self-report questionnaires. Sometimes these objective tests may give false information and it depends on honesty in reporting process of individuals. Research on psychological assessment has generally found objective tests to be more valid and reliable than projective tests.

Psychology has traditionally defined personality through its behavioral patterns, and more recently with neuroscientific studies of the brain. The introvert's behavior of actions and responses is complicated in assessing to get exact information.

PSYCHOMETRIC ASSESSMENT OF PERSONALITY

Personality is a set of individual differences that are affected by the development of an individual's values, attitudes, personal memories, social relationships, habits, and skills.

Personality assessment: Assessment implies that the consideration has been given to certain traits, values, and standards and that interpretation of the evidence has been made in the light of particular situation. The approach taken by the specialist in personality assessment is based on the assumption that much of the observable variability in behavior from one person to other results from differences in the extent to which individuals possess particular underlying personal characteristics (traits). The assessment specialist seeks to define these traits, to measure them objectively, and to relate them to socially significant aspects of behavior.

The assessment is another way of gathering information intended to know the mindset of the individual on particular subject and to increase the wise decisions to apply in their personal or professional life.

The experts of personality development introduced some techniques in observation and evaluation. Personality theorists gave prominence in their research to understand the human traits in many aspects of people's thinking, perceiving, learning, memory, etc.

Methods of Assessing Personality

- Observational method (interview)
- Personality inventories (based on trait theories)
- Projective techniques (based on psychoanalytic theories)

Personality varies from one individual to another. It is very difficult to assess exact information for evaluation.

Observational Method (Interview)

The observation methods are used on children and all ages of humans to assess their personality in different situations depending on the aim of assessment. Teacher–student relation, parent–child relation, siblings and neighborhood, etc., are considered in observational processes. These are used to evaluate a person's personality for the purpose of employment and for education as well as for identifying personality trait.

In interview method of personality assessment, the individual's general intelligence on subject matter, patience, skills, and talents may be observed by answers of related matters. The emotional levels are also noticed by feelings in complicated questions to answer. Personality tests might reveal trends that are related to his inadequate social relationships.

Questionnaires

Questionnaire is another popular method of assessment of personality by preparation of questions to conduct written or oral questions. These are used for selection of students in competitive examination from a large group of eligible candidates. Results will be declared on priority basis of scores obtained in written test. These are used in both private and public sectors in job recruitment in specific areas.

Projective Techniques (Fig. 5.13)

Based on psychoanalytic theories)

- **The Minnesota Multiphasic Personality Inventory (MMPI):** One of the most commonly used personality tests is the "Minnesota Multiphasic Personality Inventory" (MMPI). It is the most widely used multitrait scale valid for many purposes. It was started in the year 1930 to know the psychological disorders. It is also developed by simple sentenced statements in cards and booklets with minimum ability of reading. These are also used in counseling and research purpose. These are also useful to judge and compare the gathered information and personality inventory. It is also used for court cases in investigation.

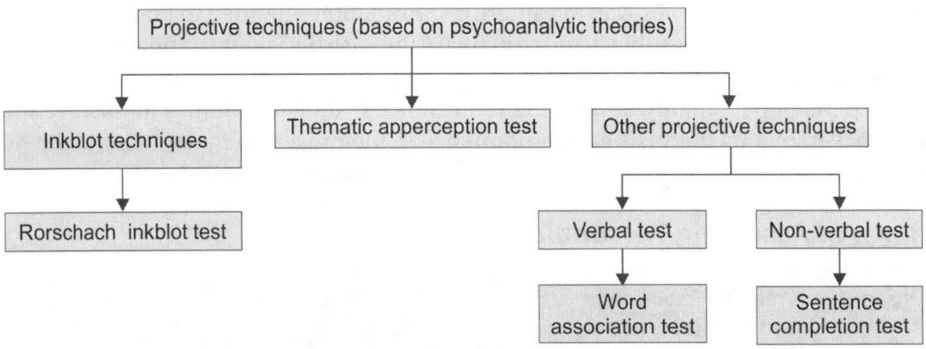

Fig. 5.13: Projective techniques

- **The Rorschach Test:** Swiss Psychologist-Hermann Rorschach **(Fig. 5.14A)** (1920) developed this test. This test is like a sample of inkblot **(Fig. 5.14B)** given below. The ink-blot test consists of 10 cards, each containing a rather elaborate inkblot **(Fig. 5.14B)**. Five blots are in color and five in gray and black. Subject studies one blot at a time and tells what each blot resembles. They can think about the inkblot as long as they like over each card. The examiner records the responses and then shows the cards a second time asking the subject to deal in detail with personal interpretation and explain which part of the blot led to their responses. There are three criteria of scoring. The complete scoring is very complex, involving many factors beyond mere counting of responses.

  Scoring whole figures shows high intelligence and ability to combine. Some forms in motion, particularly human forms, show vivid imagination; responses to color show impulsiveness and even emotional instability. Seeing animals suggests lower intelligence and nothing unusual details show introversion and mental conflicts.

  The Rorschach test consists of 10 white cards with blots of ink on them in black and red or multicolored. The individual being tested is asked to provide interpretations of the blots on the cards by stating everything that the inkblot may resemble based on their personal interpretation.

  The therapist then analyzes their responses. The idea is that unconscious needs will come out in the person's response, e.g. an aggressive person may see images of destruction.
- **The Thematic Apperception Test:** The Thematic Apperception Test (also known as the TAT) involves presenting individuals to explain the theme of pictures appearing in their mind. This information helps in assessing personality of individuals toward family and social interactions. Responses are analyzed for common themes. The responses are interpreted by unconscious feelings, thoughts, and processes. During testing, person is shown each sketch and asked to make a story about the people.

  The subject is asked to tell the examiner a story about each card that includes the following elements: the event shown in the picture **(Fig. 5.15)**; what has led up to it; what the characters in the picture are feeling and thinking; and the outcome of the event.

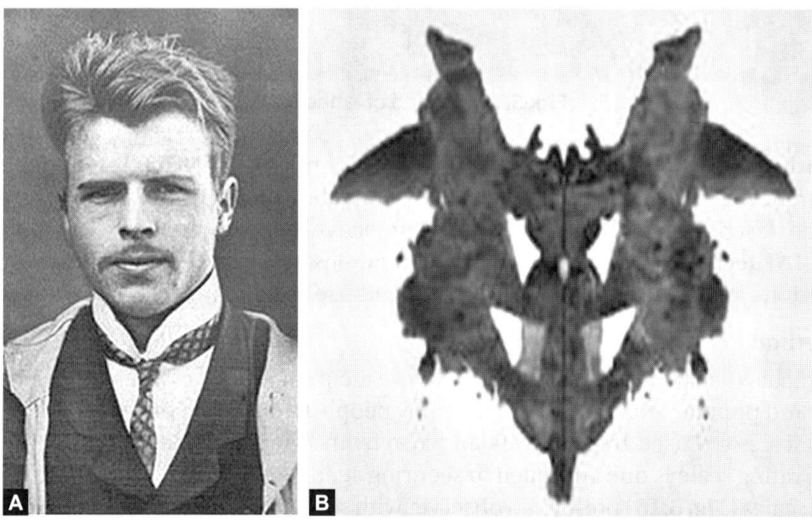

Figs. 5.14A and B: A. Hermann Rorschach (8 th Nov 1884-1st April 1922); B. Inkblot test image-1921

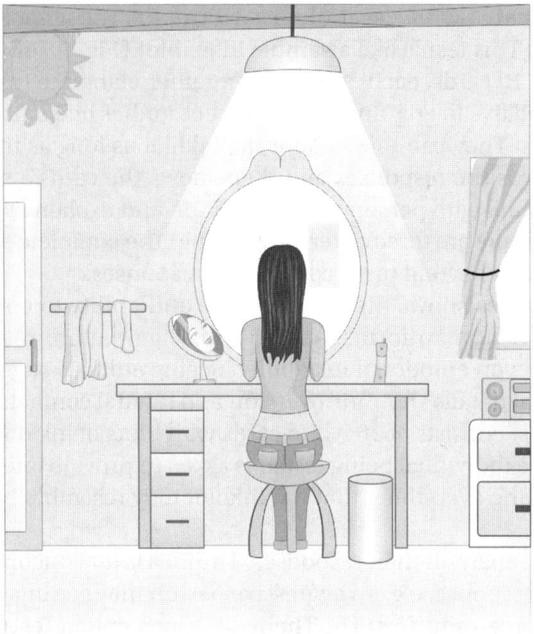

Fig. 5.15: Example for thematic apperception test

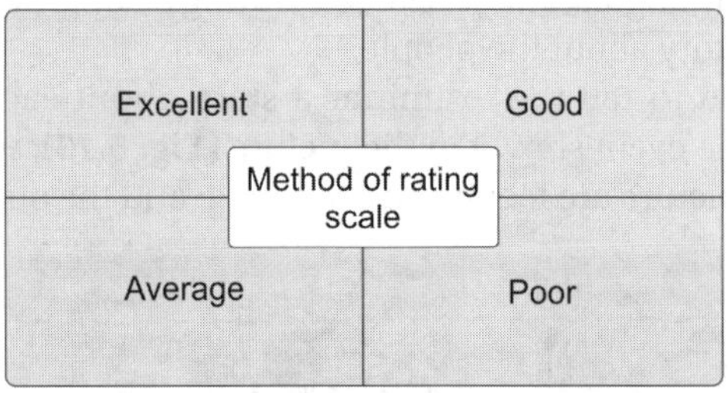

Fig. 5.16: Method of rating scale

Majority of psychologists suggested and consider not to call TAT as test better to respond right or wrong process of answering. They consider the term "technique" to be a more accurate description of the TAT and other projective assessments.

This TAT technique is useful in eliciting qualities associated with different products to perceptions about the kind of people that might use certain products or services.

Rating Method

The rating scale is common and simple projective technique in assessment of personality. It is the oldest and popular technique used by many people to know the preferences.

Rating scales are used by observers and also by individuals for self-reporting (self-report tests). The rating scale is one approach to securing such judgments..

Rating scales **(Fig. 5.16)** present an observer with scalar dimensions those who are observed are to be placed.

A teacher, for example, might be asked to rate students on the degree to which the behavior of each reflects leadership capacity, shyness, or creativity. Peers might rate each other along dimensions such as friendliness, trustworthiness, and social skills. Several standardized, printed rating scales are available for describing the behavior of psychiatric hospital patients. Relatively objective rating scales have also been devised for use with other groups. Rating scales often take a graphic form.

Personality inventories: Self-report tests—these are used to measure personality by their facial feelings while responding. They indicate personality attribution. In other words, face validity need not be defined by careful, quantitative study. It is typically reflecting one's more-or-less imprecise impressions. Self-report personality tests are used to diagnose the patient in clinical setting. These are also useful in employee's recruitment by their interest based on their attitude. It gives information to understand their anxiety and emotional levels on a particular aspect.

Eysenck personality inventory: Hans Eysenck was interested in measuring the parts (TRAITS) of a person's personality. This theory is based primarily on physiology and genetics. The behavior may be differing from one person to another by hereditary and environment factors.

A widely used early self-report inventory, the so-called Woodworth Personal Data Sheet, was developed during World War 1 to detect soldiers who were emotionally unfit for combat. Self-report question gives prominence in answering by right or wrong choice based on personal beliefs of the individuals. Rather than testing general knowledge or specific skills, personality inventories ask people questions about themselves. The subject response score is useful to identify a distinctive aspect of personality.

Computer programs: The development of computer programs is more useful in diagnosing psychological disorders of hysteria, schizophrenia, and paranoia by using MMPI responses. The most personality inventories are revised for a variety of reasons, including the need to take account of cultural and social changes and to improve them.

Word-association Techniques

In the list of projective approaches, the word association test helps in assessing personality. This type of test is easily assessing the personality in usage of words related to particular aspects and be analyzed to know the psychological status in assembling words in connection of family, social, and cultural aspects of individual personality. The investigator records the reply to each word spoken by him or her.

Sentence-completion Techniques

The sentence-completion technique is used to test of personality inventory. This is to study the attitudes, conflicts and motives of the subject. This type of analyses is similar to TAT. In most of the cases, the clinician is interested in both subjective and objective information.

Cognitive Assessment

The type of assessment depends on thoughts and feelings of the individual in personality inventory. It gives information of maladjustment and helps to the evaluator by applying the methods of questionnaire to modify the behavior of the subject. It is also developed to sample people's thoughts after an upsetting event. Beepers (electronic pagers) have been used to signal subjects to record their thoughts at certain times of the day.

Bodily Assessment

In personality inventory, bodily assessment is one of the simple methods of assessment. The subject may get bodily changes while responding to some verbal and nonverbal messages. It reveals interpretation of active, lazy, not interest to answer by different feelings, thoughts while understanding the points of evaluator.

Sophisticated devices have been developed to measure such physiological changes as pupil dilation, blood pressure, and electrical skin responses under specific conditions.

Technological advances are making it possible to monitor an individual's physiological state on a continuous basis. Sweat, heartbeat, blood volume, substances in the bloodstream, and blood pressure can all be recorded and correlated with the presence or absence of certain psychological conditions such as stress.

Alterations in Personality

Ill-health is more dangerous to continue peaceful life. The individual always tries to be sound health for well-being of physical and mental status.

The antidepressants may have a direct effect on neurochemical pathways relevant to personality, independent of changes of severe depression. They may feel insecure and not aware of recovery of their illness. The family support is more essential in crucial state of the patient.

CONCLUSION

The knowledge in understanding personality of different individuals and group will help nurse in assessment. The nurse can manage the patient acceptance for surgeries to face stressful complications. The knowledge of personality tests and projective techniques helps in estimating the interest, skills, and abilities in understanding human personality. The nurse has to manage patients of different age groups in her profession. The convincing attitude of nurse by study of personality development in psychology to get success in both personal and professional life.

QUESTIONS

Essay Questions

1. Explain the theories of personality. Discuss the various trait components necessary to have effective nurse-patient relationship.
2. Define personality. Explain the topography and dynamic aspects of mind.
3. Define personality. Explain Freud's Psychoanalytic theory.

Short Notes

1. Describe the personality changes that occur in individual. How does it influence the field of nursing practice?
2. Define personality and discuss any one type.
3. Explain one theory of personality.
4. Freud theory of personality.
5. Types of personality tests.

Brief Questions

1. Psychological assessment of personality.
2. Projective technique.
3. Rorschach inkblot test.
4. Superego.
5. Introverts.
6. Expand TAT.
7. Rating method.
8. List the types of personality.
9. List the salient features of topography of personality.
11. Difference between ego and super ego.
12. Define extrovert.

Fill in the Blanks

1. The term personality is derived from the Latin word ______ which means "mask." (persona)
2. Extrovert, introvert, and ambivert were proposed by ______ classification-based on sociability. (Carl Jung)
3. According to Sigmund Freud's psychoanalytic theory, three structural elements of personality id, ______, and superego. (ego)
4. Ego is the ______ (reality principle).
5. Freud's three levels of consciousness are unconscious, preconscious and ______ (consciousness).
6. ______ classified the personality based on psycho-sexual development of the individual four stages—oral, anal, phallic, and genital. (Sigmund Freud)
7. Thematic ______ test (TAT) is a projective technique. (apperception)
8. Minnesota ______ personality inventory. (multiphasic)
9. The Rorschach inkblot test is also one of the ______ techniques of personality. (projective)

Multiple Choice Questions

1. The term personality comes from the ....
   a. German word
   b. Greek word
   c. Latin word
2. Extrovert, introvert and ambivert were proposed by ....
   a. Eysenck
   b. Carl Jung
   c. Sheldon
3. Endomorphic, mesomorphic and ectomorphic classification was proposed by ....
   a. Galton
   b. Eysenck
   c. Sheldo

4. Projective techniques are ....
   a. Thematic Apperception test
   b. Sentence completion test
   c. Both
5. The screening device of a personality test is ....
   a. MMPI
   b. CAT
   c. TAT

Answers

1. c	2. b	3. c	4. c	5. a

CHAPTER 6

Developmental Psychology

Learning Objectives

- Developmental psychology
- Psychology of people at different ages from infancy to old age
- Psychology of vulnerable individuals—challenged, women, sick, etc.
- Psychology of groups

Developmental psychology explains the changes occurred in human growth from birth till death. Developmental psychologists try to understand complex behavior by studying their beginning and in orderly ways which they change or develop over the lifespan. It depends on past experiences, genes, and environmental conditions of human life.

It focus upon development during childhood, adolescence, adulthood, and old age. Developmental psychologists also study on a wide range of theoretical areas, such as biological, social, emotion, and cognitive processes. In 1980, researchers of Japan concentrated more in this field.

Finally, developmental psychologists hope to optimize development, and apply their theories to help people in practical situations (e.g., help parents develop secure attachments with their children).

Definitions

The human being is never static from conception to death. Development means "a progressive series of changes that occur in an orderly predictable pattern as a result of maturation and experience".

The branch developmental psychology studies physical, cognitive, and social changes throughout the lifespan. It brings awareness of goals and values in modifying human behavior to reach their destinations.

DEVELOPMENT OF PSYCHOLOGY OF PEOPLE AT DIFFERENT AGES (INFANCY TO OLD AGE)

The industrial growth gave more prominence to study developmental psychology in workforce, stress, emotional levels, etc. Some other causes depend on childhood experiences of family, education, and social aspects of the individual.

Theories of Developmental Psychology

Evolutionary Developmental Psychology

Charles Darwin in 1877 published a paper with details on development of innate forms of communication based on scientific observations of his infant son, Doddy. He was the first person who conducted systematic study of developmental psychology.

Charles Darwin applied basic principles on natural selection in Theory of Evolution. Darwin gave importance to environment in social and cognitive development of the individual.

Later in 1882, another German physiologist, Wilhelm Preyer published a book based on specific discipline "The Mind of the Child".

In 1900, some other theorists dominated the field with their extensive theories of human development, Jean Piaget (1896–1980), Lev Vygotsky (1896–1934) and John Bowlby (1907–1990).

Cognitive Development

Jean Piaget explained that the moral development is different in children **(Fig. 6.1)** compared to adults. Each child may be different from another.

Expanding on Piaget's work, Lawrence Kohlberg determined that the process of moral development was principally concerned with justice, and that it continued throughout the individual's lifetime.

Most of these theorists explained all these from their personal lives of family members.

Lev Vygotsky **(Fig. 6.2)** was a Russian theorist from the Soviet era, who posited that children learn through hands-on experience and social interactions with members of his/her culture.

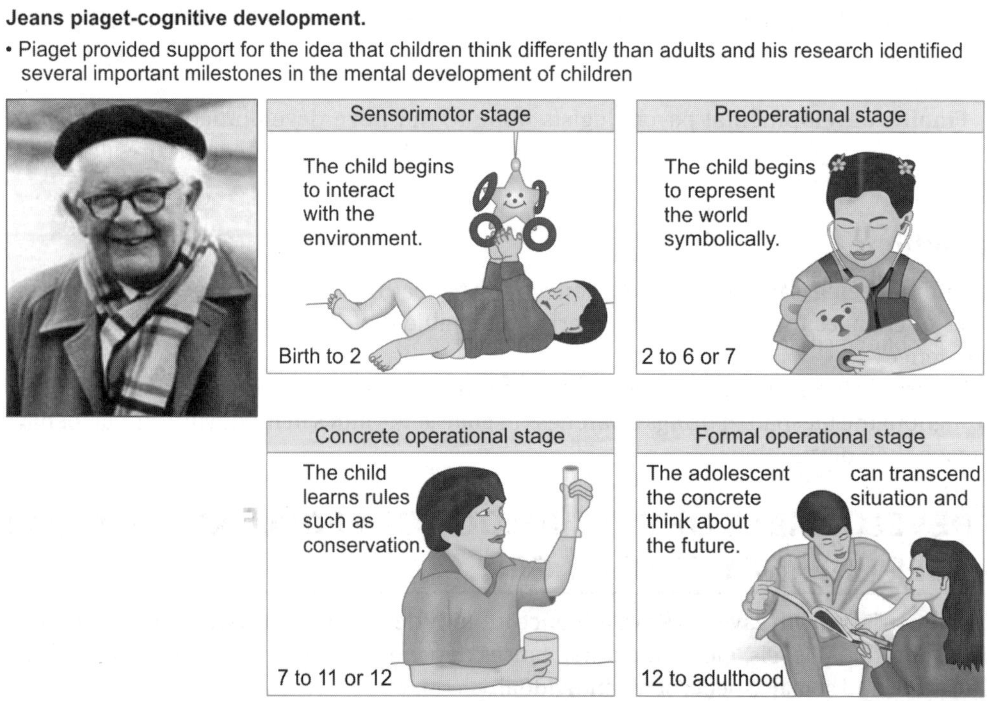

Fig. 6.1: Jean Piaget stage of cognitive development

Vygotsky's theories stress the fundamental role of social interaction in the development of cognition.

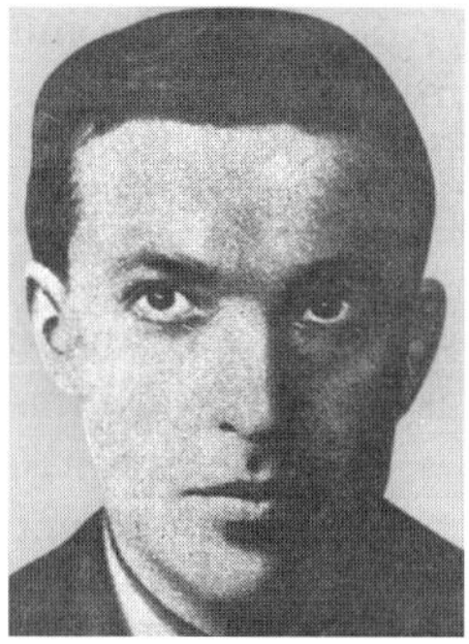

Fig. 6.2: Lev Vygotsky

Attachment Theory of Development

He was the first attachment theorist, describing attachment as a lasting psychological connectedness between human beings.

According to Bowlby **(Fig. 6.3A)**, attachment developed in children by providing basic necessities for survival. Bowlby described attachment as a biological system of support of warm, intimate, and close relations from mother to infants to face impulses in improvement of their survival. It is also associated with emotional bonds of children.

Attachment feeds on body contact and familiarity **(Fig. 6.3B).** It forms basis of personality development and socialization (evolutionary and biological significance).

Psychosexual Development

Sigmund Freud believed there is tension between the conscious and unconscious because the conscious tries to hold back what the unconscious tries to express. Freud developed three personality structures which are id functions on pleasure principle, ego on realistic, and super-ego stands on morality. Based on this, Freud proposed four universal stages in personality development. It is the source of the child's psychosexual energy **(Table 6.1)**.

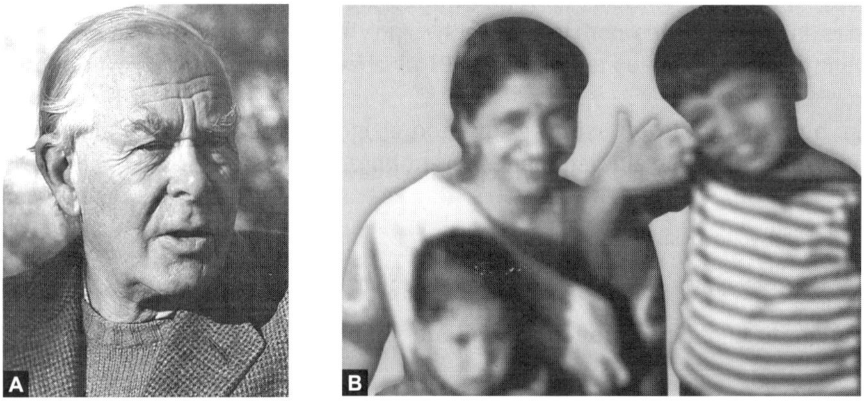

Figs. 6.3A and B: (A) John Bowlby; (B) Example for attachment theory

Table 6.1: Stages of psychosexual development

S. no.	*Stage*	*Age group*	*Erogenous zone*
1.	Oral	0 to 8 months	Mouth
2.	Anal	18 months to 3 years	Bowl and bladder elimination
3.	Phallic	3 to 5 years	Genital
4.	Latent	6 years to puberty	Sexual interest mature
5.	Genital	Puberty to death	Matured sexual interest

Some developmental psychologists studied developmental change covering the lifespan from conception to death **(Fig. 6.4)**. Among the different developmental psychologists, the views presented by Erickson and Havighurst appear to give a comprehensive picture of development of human individual from infancy to old age.

Erik Erickson (1902–1994) was a student of Sigmund Freud. He offered a modified Freudian view of development of personality **(Table 6.2)**. He gave importance to social and cultural aspects of development of personality.

According to Erikson, the developmental task arises in individual in certain period.

The development of psychology is classified into different stages in human growth.

Infancy, childhood, adolescence, adulthood, and old-age.

Infancy (Birth to 18 months): This stage covers early days after birth, nearly two weeks of life. It is oral stage. The development is very short in this level. The new born infant must make four major adjustments to postnatal life. The child has to adjust to the changes of temperature from mother's womb to outside of it.

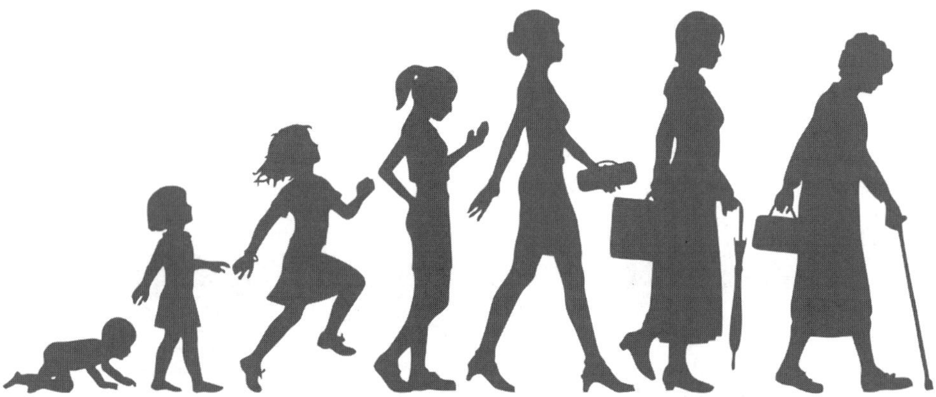

Fig. 6.4: Stage of proximal development

Table 6.2: Erikson psychosocial development

Childhood	Trust vs. mistrust	Faith in the environment and future environment	Suspicious, fear of future events
	Autonomy vs. doubt	A sense of self-control and adequacy	Feelings of shame and self-doubt
	Initiative vs. guilt	Ability to be a "self-starter," to initiate one's own activities	A self of inadequacy to be on one's own
	Industry vs. inferiority	Ability to learn how things work, to understand and organize	A sense of inferiority at understanding and organizing
Adolescence	Identity vs. confusion	Seeing oneself as a unique and integrated person	Confusion over who and what one really is
Adulthood	Intemacy vs isolation	Ability to make commitments to others, to love	Inability to form affectionate relationships
Old age	Integrity vs. despair	A sense of integrity and fulfillment, willingness to face death	Dissatisfaction with life, despair over prospect of death

The infant may feel difficulty in early hours of birth and slowly adjusts to new atmosphere. The infant may struggle to fulfill hunger drive by breast feeding (sucking), swallowing, and elimination.

This period extends from birth to 18 months of age. This is called the age of trust vs. mistrust.

Trust versus Mistrust

The infant who comes to the new environment from mother's womb needs only nourishment. The baby responds to noises and other stimuli. The infant may feel discomfort in adjustment. The caregivers provide attention toward infants in every second of early 18 months while learning new tasks of crawling, sitting, standing, and in imitation creates trust in them. Thus, a child cannot learn to walk or toilet training without the support of mother or caregivers.

In this period, child observes the attention of mother and family members who are assisting them in learning process which gives clarity on trust. The infant learns to trust others and develops confidence. It provides affection and love toward them and expectations from them in fulfilling their desires. If the infant fails to get attention from caregivers, it causes mistrust which affects the personality in later stages of life.

- **Toddler:** This stage ranges from 18 months to 3 years.
- **Autonomy versus shame**: The child learns new tasks by imitation of family members, friends, and neighborhood. The children try to solve their problems by managing friendly relations. The child needs guidance. It is called autonomy vs. shame. The child takes solids in this age and eliminates body wastes. He tries to speak openly in the presence of family members and others. The child develops doubt about its abilities. The child attends to school by learning all these and tries to adjust with classmates.

  The child's needs and environmental factors, requires the caretaker's careful and constant attention.
- **Preschool:** This stage extends from 3years to 5 years.
- **Initiative versus guilt:** The child will begin to imitate the parents of the same sex and unconsciously wish to replace that parent in the family. The caretaker recognizes recognizes that the child's creative effort in attempting to do some activities is encouraged, the crisis will be resolved in favorable direction and this outcome, if repeated, should influence the future initiative. Otherwise, the child develops feelings of guilt.

  During this period, the little boy who always had a great deal of attention and love from his mother begins to feel very possessive toward the mother. He develops competitive feelings toward his father and tries to gain mother's love. Similarly, the girl wants to gain father's attention toward her and tries to develop competitive spirit in gaining attention of father toward her instead of their mother.
- **School age:** This period ranges from 5 years to 12 years.
- **Industry versus inferiority:** During this period, child develops interest toward opposite sex. In latency stage, child suffers insufficient sleep by fantasy. The child wants spare life with peer group to share their feelings and thoughts. He develops skills which are useful to compete and cooperate in getting success in his future. The child develops sense of industry verses inferiority. The failure of tasks makes him to feel inferior in the presence of elders.
- **The adolescence (Teens):** This period is from 12 years to 20 years.

  It is called as transition period; many changes occur in this age in both genders. It is puberty period for sexual, social, and emotional changes in human behavior.

  Stanley Hall has rightly described this period as **a "period of storm and stress".**

- **The role confusion/identity confusion:** The boys and girls get attraction to opposite sex. The adolescence is newly concerned with how he or she appears to others. The children develop a sense of sexual identity.

  It is a turning point in human life; by following good guidance, he will develop a sense of self or identity which makes him a good human being. The wrong guidance or indiscipline makes him to suffer from role confusion/identity confusion.
- **The adulthood:** The early adulthood extends from 20 years to 30 years.
- **Intimacy versus isolation:** The new responsibilities can create tensions and frustrations, and one solution involved is an intimate relationship with family. This situation leads to a crisis called intimacy vs. isolation.

  The adults also deeply think to choose life partner to share his feelings of love and affection. Sometimes isolations lead to conflicts and frustrations. The unemployment may lead to suffering economic problems.

  The later adulthood starts from 30 years to 65 years. Most of the people face difficulties in managing family, adjustment to life-partner, supporting old parents, taking care of new entries in family, and managing finances for well and healthy being of the family. This stage is called generativity vs. stagnation. If this goal is not achieved, the individual will be disappointed and experience a feeling of stagnation.
- **The old age:** The old age starts after 65 years. Most of the people in this age want to settle down the issues of family and try to plan for rest in this period.
- **The integrity versus despair:** The crisis in this stage is the integrity vs. despair in which the person finds meaning in memories or instead looks back on life with dissatisfaction. There is lack of strength, physical energy, and decreased income, sometimes death of spouse and unfulfilled desires lead to decline of health.

PSYCHOLOGY OF VULNERABLE INDIVIDUALS—CHALLENGED, WOMEN, SICK, ETC.

According to South African Concise Oxford dictionary, "Vulnerable" originated from the Latin term "vulnerare," which means "to wound." Dictionary meaning of vulnerable: "exposed to being attacked or harmed, either physically or emotionally."

The vulnerability of individuals is extended to race, ethnicity, age, gender, and other causes to feel weak for their progress. Vulnerable groups are classified into three categories.

The defects in physical growth are one of the risk factors for infants and sick group. The chronic conditions, respiratory problems, diabetes, hypertension, and heart diseases also may cause vulnerability.

Managing mentally retarded and providing mental recovery are difficult tasks to family members. It is of high risk to control the chronic patient without the support of psychiatrist or clinical psychologist. The isolation and addiction for alcohol and drugs may lead to suicidal tendencies in individuals.

The social circumstances lead to another type of vulnerability; for example: Poverty, unemployment, illiteracy, caste system, racial and ethnic minorities, and maladjustment etc. Superstitions in orthodox families are also one of the social domains of vulnerability.

In late childhood, children are not strong compared to elders. The physical handicap is also another drawback to fulfill their desires of completing tasks. It causes for difficulty in motor and sensory activities.

Some other social factors of vulnerability in children are broken families, step-parents, ill treatment, and poverty. It gives chance of isolation and depressed life in children. Disability, emotional problems, substance use, direct experience of physical or sexual violence, and severe chronic illness are also causes of vulnerability **(Fig 6.5)**.

Some other factors of vulnerability in girl children **(Fig. 6.6)** are negligence and gender partialities among the parents and other family members. Discouragement of education, employment, and lack of freedom are also social domains of vulnerability in girl children.

With an estimated 12.6 million children engaged in hazardous occupations (2001 Census), for instance, India has the largest number of child laborers under the age of 14 in the world. Among children, there are some groups like street children and children of sex workers who face additional forms of discrimination. A large number of children are reportedly trafficked to the neighboring countries. Trafficking of children also continues to be a serious problem in India.

National girl child day celebration was started by the Women and Child Development Ministry in 2008.

The aims of these programs are to bring awareness on gender equality, importance to female literacy, legal rights, medical care, and protection from discrimination. It is also aimed to eradicate child marriages and violence to women.

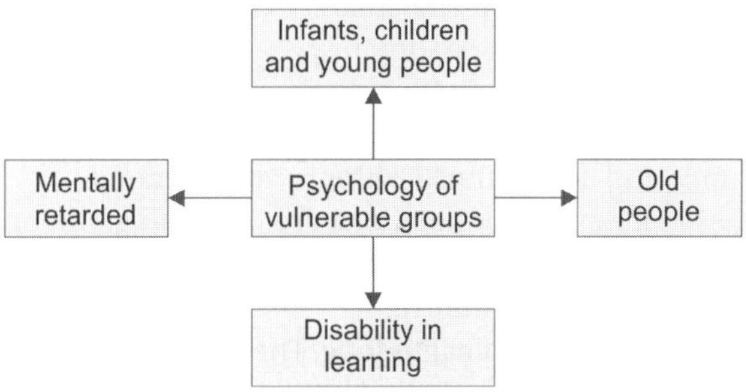

Fig. 6.5: Health domains of vulnerable populations

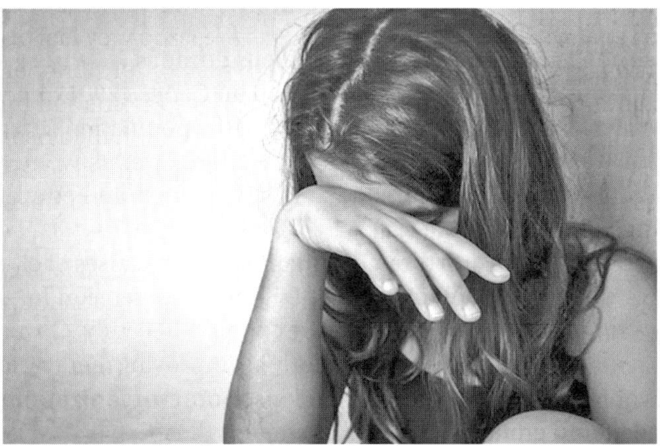

Fig. 6.6: Vulnerability in children

Women

The vulnerability of women and sick is connected to the inability to cope with day-to-day life. The women are vulnerable in pregnancy, in early days after delivery, menstrual disorders, etc. This situation affects different aspects of an individual's life—which may be physical, psychological, social, spiritual, or developmental in nature.

Some women face problems such as marital problems, dowry harassment, sexual harassment, and gender inequalities in working areas. It creates psychological disturbance, depression, and frustration and even leads to suicidal deaths.

In India, the average maternal mortality ratio at national level is 540 deaths per 100,000 live births (National Family Health Survey-2, 2000).

The rural MMR (maternal mortality death) is 617 deaths of women aged between 15 and 49 years per one lakh live births (NFHS 2000).

Sick

The thought of severe sickness may reduce hopes in life, which leads to depression in sick group. The burden of managing family, children, and old parents also causes frustrating moments for sick. It reduces lifespan.

For example, the number of uninsured patients younger than 65 years of age grew by nearly 6 million between 2000 and 2004, with the greatest growth in those who are poor (46%) or near-poor (22%). In this population, approximately 35–45% have at least one chronic medical condition. More than half (58%) of those with a chronic illness without insurance reported that they did not buy a prescription drug in 2003 because of cost compared with 39% of those with publicly funded insurance and 34% of those with private insurance.

The numbers of these vulnerable populations are increasing, not only as the ranks of the uninsured grow, but as the population ages. Some of the health conditions make him to depend on others and make him to become handicap.

Disabilities are another barrier to suffer life-long. They suffer for food, psychological support, and other basic needs. It creates tensions and irrational fears in leading life. In India, nearly 21.9 million people are suffering with disabilities. 2.13% of disabled population are suffering.

Elderly

In India, elderly was not a vulnerable group in previous decades.

According to data on the age of India's population, in Census 2001, there were a little over 76.6 million people above 60 years, constituting 7.2% of the population. The number of people over 60 years in 1991 was 6.8% of the country's population. Overall, women in 45 to 64 years of age who are unemployed and uninsured with lower incomes and education levels tend to report the poorest health status **(Table 6.3)**.

The death of spouse, poverty, and drought situation are the causes of elderly as vulnerable. The isolation, migration, and lack of love and attention create tension in elderly. The lack of psychological support reduces the life span in our country. Recently, Government supported special schemes to reduce the vulnerability in elderly by improving medical facilities, insurance schemes, and traveling benefits to senior citizens. Some organizations provide special opportunities to the retired group.

Table 6.3: The number of disabilities in India in 2002

Disability Data as per National Survey Organization (NSSO) 2002	
Disability	*Percentage among total population*
Movement	51%
Seeing	14%
Hearing	15%
Speech	10%
Mental	10%

Mentally Retarded

The chronic illness and prolonged disability make the person feel anger on him and on others. They need the support of relationships to recover from vulnerability. The psychological support is more essential for mentally retarded. The proper attention of love and affection in family and economic support are important aspects to reduce the mentally retarded.

The lack of awareness on psychological disorders is the main cause of vulnerability. At primary level, depression, distress, isolation, and other psychological disturbances can be solved by counseling.

Eighty-seven percent of those of 65 years and older have one or more chronic conditions, and 67% of this population have two or more chronic illnesses.

The strength of psychologists, clinical psychologists, and psychiatrists in the country can reduce the vulnerability of mentally retarded.

Mental Health Act drafted by Parliament in 1987 replaced the Indian Lunacy Act in 1912.

Sexual Minorities

The sexual minorities are identified as gay and hijra. The discrimination of these creates inferiority among this group. Individuals who are identified as having the same-sex sexual preferences are ridiculed and ostracized by their own family and are left with very limited support structures and networks of community that provide them conditions of care and support. Their needs and concerns are excluded from the various health policies and programs. In recent days, these are also forming groups to solve their problems with the support of Government.

India declares freedom of sexual orientation a fundamental right. "Discrimination against an individual on the basis of sexual orientation is deeply offensive to the dignity and self-worth of the individual."

The stress-related problems are increased in sexual minorities due to stigma. In sexual minority group, behavioral changes of stigma lead to problems of coping regulation, social and cognitive process, and risk factors of psychopathology.

PSYCHOLOGY OF GROUPS

The group is an important process in managing healthy social relations of society.

WE Bogardus defined that the term group refers to "number of units of anything to close proximity with one another."

MacIver and Page said a group refers to "any collection of human beings, brought into social relationships with one another."

These are also useful in learning, working, problem solving, and planning of major projects in day-to-day life. The group activity is an essential activity in every path of life. The individual's behavior is entirely different when he is in group. The addiction therapies of alcoholism and drug addiction are treated by group therapies.

Group Structure

In structure of group, two or more are necessary to form a group. The forming of group is based on purpose and role of the member and managing group activities. The responsibility is an important process in achieving goal and social interactions in every level of the process.

There are mainly two types of groups:

1. Primary groups
2. Secondary groups.

Primary Groups

CH Cooley "by primary group meant "those characterized by intimate face to face association and cooperation. They are primary in several senses, but chiefly they are fundamental informing social-nature and ideals of the individual." For example, Family, friends, etc.

Primary groups are also the key means of socialization in society, the main place where attitudes, values, and orientations are developed and sustained.

Secondary Groups

According to Cooley, "Secondary groups are wholly lacking in intimacy of association and usually in most of the other primary and quasi-primary characteristics." E.g.: State, University, Trade unions, etc.

The secondary groups are large in size and usually formally organized. They are an important place for socialization, but secondary to primary groups.

The Psychological Significance of Groups

The people are capable to live alone, but they prefer to be in company by sharing the values, problems in social interaction. They may get solution to several issues and feel pleasure leading life in group.

The Group Affiliation in Groups

The group interaction may provide support in solving major projects by role of different members to face the challenges by assistance, cooperation, and group discussion for both psychological and social support in all levels of their process. It is responsibility of each individual in the team to accept with group norms.

Leon Festinger's Theory of Social Comparison (1950, 1954) suggested that in many cases people join with others to evaluate the accuracy of their personal beliefs and attitudes.

Stanley Schachter (1959) explored this process by putting individuals in ambiguous, stressful situations and asking them if they wished to wait alone or with others.

Individuals in groups can secure advantages and avoid disadvantages by their interest in adjusting to different people in the groups.

A group may include many talented individuals, but they must learn how to pool their individual abilities and energies to maximize the team's performance. In team work, success depends on coordination from all sides of direction in reaching destination. They may face barriers or frustration in getting solutions. The noncooperation leads to failure in reaching targets.

Social loafing can be a problem because one way to overcome it is by recognizing that each group member has an important part to play in the success of the group.

Group Dynamics

Group dynamics is a system of behaviors and psychological processes. The choice in choosing leaders, allotting work is based on talent, leadership qualities, impartial of caste system, racism, gender inequalities, personal interest in purpose of success, and peaceful atmosphere in achievement. These applications of the field are studied in psychology, sociology, anthropology, political science, epidemiology, education, social work business, and communication studies.

In the modern society, most of the recruitment is getting support of psychologists to deal with behavior. Groups not only generate more ideas and possible solutions by discussing the problem, but they can also more objectively evaluate the options that they generate during discussion.

CONCLUSION

The view of adjustment and dynamics influences on reciprocity between children and family. Developmental psychology helps nurses in understanding emotional, intellectual thoughts, feelings, and attitudes. It gives special guidance in adjusting with patients of different age groups to diagnose and treatment. The knowledge of developmental psychology helps nurses to deal the patients in group therapies of addiction and drugs. The awareness of the psychology of vulnerable may help nurses in understanding their weakness in social adjustment and other complicated situations. The special knowledge on psychology of social groups helps nurses in health awareness of development of community projects in immunization programs and prevention of infectious diseases. It also helps nurses in changing superstitions and beliefs in rural communities.

QUESTIONS

Essay Questions

1. What do you mean by group of psychology? Describe psychology of people of different ages.
2. Discuss the behavioral changes that occur in stages from infancy to old age.

Short Notes

1. Vulnerable groups.
2. Psychological development during adolescence.
3. Explain the stages of development.
4. Describe psychological needs of patients.
5. Assessment of personality.
6. Explain psychological needs of women.

Brief Questions

1. Geriatric problems.
2. Psychological needs of women.
3. Explain the psychology of adolescence.
4. Enumerate the types of developmental psychology.
5. List any four features of psychology of sick people.

Fill in the Blanks

1. Developmental psychology explains the changes occur in ____________ from birth till death. (human growth)
2. Freud proposed four universal stages in personality development of child's psychosexual energy—oral stage, ____________, phallic stage, and genital stage. (anal stage)
3. ____________ called as transition period as many changes occur in this age in both genders. It is puberty period for sexual, social, and emotional changes in human behavior. (adolescence)
4. Infants, children, and sick are called as ____________ group. (vulnerable)

Multiple Choice Questions

1. Autonomy vs shame and doubt is seen in ....
   a. Infancy
   b. Toddler
   c. School age child
2. Intimacy vs isolation is seen in ....
   a. Young adulthood
   b. Adolescence
   c. Late adulthood
3. Sigmund freud psychosexual development stages ....
   a. Anal
   b. Oral
   c. Both

Answers

1. b	2. a	3. c

CHAPTER 7

Mental Hygiene and Mental Health

Learning Objectives

- Concepts of mental hygiene and mental health
- Characteristics of mentally healthy person
- Warning signs of poor mental health
- Promote and prevent mental health—strategies and services
- Ego-defence mechanisms and implications
- Personal and social adjustments
- Guidance and counseling
- Role of nurse

ORIGIN OF THE MENTAL HYGIENE MOVEMENT

The National Committee for Mental Hygiene was founded in New York in 1909. Many of the researchers planned to improve medical facilities for the mentally retarded people with the powers of nation.

Mental hygiene originated from the branch of psychiatry in medicine.

During 1920, Sigmund Freud's psychoanalytic ideas emphasized the importance of early childhood experiences and their effects on mental health. Most of the mental illness can be prevented by proper medical care in early days of the problems. Preventive intervention is better than to face it in crucial stages. The mental hygienists also emphasized the importance of therapeutic intervention for highly emotional individuals.

CONCEPTS OF MENTAL HYGIENE AND MENTAL HEALTH

The concept of mental health is an old one, but has become popular in modern days due to awareness on this concept. In ancient days, although the cause of mental disease could be identified, the cure from the disease was difficult and not well known.

The concept of mental hygiene and mental health also depends on both physical and mental status of the individual. The healthy life of the individual depends on proper functioning of body and mind coordination. The balancing of emotions, social adjustment by maintaining harmony in both personal and social life is an art of living.

The process of mental hygiene depends on fulfilling of desires in reaching goals and making individual to lead life with both personal and social adjustment. It depends on managing emotions and balancing stress levels of human behavior.

A person faces success and failures in his day-to-day life by the process of facing emotional situations, negative feelings, getting solutions, etc. The negative thoughts of fear, jealousy, and anger lead to depressive status in mental health. Modification of behavior from fearful thoughts, feelings, depressions, severe frustrations, and conflicts causes weak and unhealthy development of personality in human beings. The long duration of this process affects both physical and psychological health of the individual.

Mental hygiene is a science study or process for healthy psychological behavior, preventing mental disorders in healthy development of personality of human beings. Mental hygiene includes all measures taken to promote and to preserve mental health by using some defense mechanisms in day-to-day life.

Definitions

WHO definition of health: "A state of complete physical, mental, and social well-being and not merely the absence of disease or infirmity."

Mental hygiene: Mental hygiene consists of measures to reduce the incidence of mental illness through prevention and early treatment and to promote mental health. Singh and Tiwari-1971.

Mental hygiene: According to Klien, "Mental hygiene is an endeavor to aid people to ward off trouble as well as to furnish ways of handling trouble in intelligent fashion when it cannot be warded off".

Mental hygiene: "It is organized attempt to effect human adjustment through the application of principles and practices of living". Bhatia BD and M Craig.

Mental Health and Mental Illness

According to the US surgeon general (1999), mental health is successful performance of mental function, resulting in productive activities, fulfilling relationships with other people, and providing the ability to adapt a change and cope with adversity.

The term mental illness refers collectively to all diagnosable mental disorders—health conditions characterized by alterations in thinking, mood, or behavior associated with distress or impaired functioning.

The term **mental health** is closely related with the term mental hygiene as the main objective of mental hygiene is to attain mental health.

Mental health is defined as "A state of well-being in which every individual realizes his or her own potential, can cope with normal stress of life, can work productively and fruitfully, and is able to make a contribution to his or her community."

Mental health: "Simultaneous success at working, loving and creating with the capacity for mature and flexible resolution of conflicts between instincts, conscience, important other people, and reality" (The American Psychiatric Association,1980).

Mental illness: "Mentally ill person means who is in need of treatment by reason of any mental disorder other than mental retardation" (Indian Mental Health/1987).

In ancient days, the lack of awareness about mental illness in public was main drawback and cause of severe mental illness. They struggled with a lot of depression, frustration, and social maladjustment due to their mental illness. Some of the depressed people used to take alcohol, drugs, and drugs to forget their sorrowful situations in their life for survival. It became a serious problem than cancer or heart diseases. Evidence from the World Health Organization (WHO) suggests that nearly half of the world's population is affected by mental illness with an impact on their self-esteem, relationships, and ability in human behavior.

Differences between Mentally Healthy and Mentally Unhealthy (Table 7.1)

The good mental health helps in progress of healthy personality development. The people who are suffering and experiencing depression, anxiety, grief, addiction, anxiety, and mood disorders are not having awareness toward healthy development of personality. Counseling members, clinical psychologists, and psychiatrists can avoid the severity in it. It helps to face the challenges toward the psychological disturbances in their life.

Several Factors Affecting Mental Health (Fig. 7.1)

The biological and psychological conditions influence human behavior in mental health. It depends on several factors of heredity, social environment of family, culture, customs, and tradition. The economic condition of unemployment and lack of resources causes psychological disturbance and social maladjustment. It leads to mental disorder of individuals.

Types of Mental Illness

Different conditions in life are recognized as mental illness.

- **Anxiety:** These types of people get easily upset by severe sweating, raise of heart beat, and feel of phobias.

Table 7.1: Differences between mentally healthy and mentally unhealthy

	Mentally healthy	*Mentally unhealthy*
1.	Mentally healthy person is able to make adjustment	Mentally unhealthy person feels discomfort in adjustment
2.	He is emotionally balanced in stressful situations	He may be disturbed by imbalance of emotions, frustration, and conflicts
3.	Mentally healthy person is effective in coping skills	Distress situation of excess fear, anxiety, and worry appears in these people's behavior
4.	Capable of taking wise decisions by social interactions and can use all types of techniques for well-being in their life	Lack of efforts in decision-making and feel alone, incapable of managing stressful situations in day-to-day life
5.	Good in managing relations of family, friends, etc.	The mentally unhealthy person is not interested in social interactions and needs loneliness

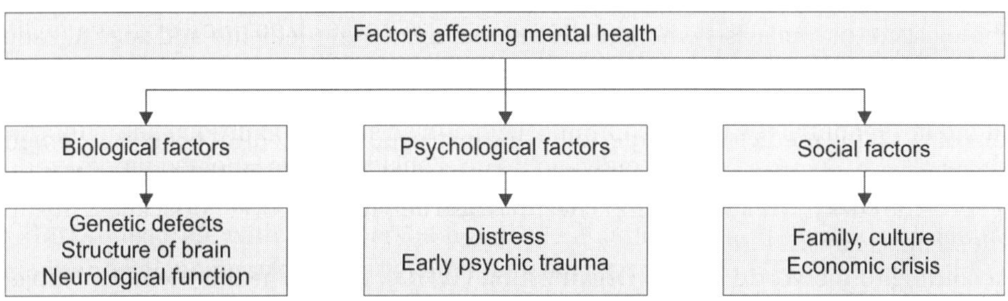

Fig. 7.1: Affecting factors of mental disorder

- **Mood disorders:** Some of the disorders of mood need loneliness. They will express irritations for simple reason and silent atmosphere. Behavior is flexible. The most common mood disorders are depressions and bipolar disorders.
- **Psychotic disorder:** The symptoms of psychological disorders are abnormal in perception like unexpected fears, imagining horror situation, sounds, disturbed sleep, etc. There is no peace of mind. Schizophrenia is an example of a psychotic disorder.
- **Distress:** It is negative stress. The distress leads to depression and frustration. It depends on physiological, psychological, and social conditions of the individual. Its extremes lead to severe mental illness.
- **Personality disorders**: The crisis of finance and lack of family support lead to anti-social behavior to satisfy his desires by addiction of alcohol and drugs to lead life.
- **Obsessive-compulsive disorder (OCD):** The disturbing thoughts are called obsessions, and the rituals are called compulsions.
- **Sexual and gender disorders:** These include disorders that affect sexual desire, performance, and behavior. Sexual dysfunction and gender identity disorder are examples of sexual and gender difference .

  One or more somatic symptoms that are distressing cause disruption in daily life.

  People with somatic symptom disorder refuse to believe their symptoms of irrational and emotional causes rather than physical causes.
- **Dementia**: Dementia is a syndrome, not a disease. The World Health Organization says that 47.5 million people around the world are living with dementia.

Parkinson's Disease Dementia

The changes in brain caused by Parkinson's disease begin in a region that plays a key role in movement. The changes in brain by Parkinson's disease gradually spread and affect mental function.

In a survey conducted by Central Health and Family Ministry of India 2014, 1 person out of every 20 suffered with stress and depression; 13.7% suffered with other mental problems in our country; people in 20 to 35 years age group suffered with professional stress. Approximately 5 crores mentally ill patients from Indian population.

Mental Health

Mental health is attaining psychological well-being. It means that both body and mind are working efficiently and harmoniously. Physical health is also associated with mental health by taking nutritious food, good sleep, body fitness, etc. The mental ill-health is treated by clinical psychologists or psychiatrists who got educational degree in medicine and specialization in clinical psychology or psychiatry. The physicians provide treatment to the physical sickness. Physicians can observe the general process in treatment and cooperation of the patient for treatment by taking medicines in time, following instructions of medical team, etc. Sometimes the physician needs the support of family members in diagnosing the patient for speedy recovery of the client. The sound mental health is also helpful in recovery of sickness by support of general physicians.

According to the World Health Organization (WHO), mental health includes "subjective well-being, perceived self-efficacy, autonomy, competence, inter-generational dependence, and self-actualization of one's intellectual and emotional potential, among others". The

WHO further states that the well-being of an individual is encompassed in the realization of their abilities, coping with normal stresses of life, productive work, and contribution to their community.

A widely accepted definition of health by mental health specialists and psychoanalyst Sigmund Freud is: the capacity "to work and to love."

Characteristics of Mental Health

Different authors emphasized different characteristics of a mentally healthy person.

> ➢ **Indian views:** Indian concept of mental health is available in the Atharva Veda which provides detailed information on mental disorder and their treatment. According to Atharva Veda, mental personality consists of three gunas or characteristics: Sattya, Rajas, and Tamas. The imbalance of these gunas causes mental disorder.
>
> These points are connected to mind from birth and balance the behavior of the individual.
>
> **The Charak Samhita** and **Susrut** have also given the concept of mental health, but they do not differ significantly from the Atharva Veda's concept of mental health.
>
> ➢ **Western concept:** Though the concept of mental health is comparatively new, different authors have given different views regarding sound mental health. Harry Stack Sullivaa says that a mentally healthy individual would place a major value on efficient social functioning.

Sigmund Freud emphasized on level of unconsciousness to motivate or control the behavior of human being.

Jahoda (1963) proposed six criteria of the mentally healthy individual.

- Mentally healthy person can handle the relationship efficiently according to his requirement and problem solution.
- The individual perceives reality in sensitive and empathetic view.
- The mentally healthy person can manage and balance stress levels in healthy way.
- Capable of decision-making.
- Growth, self-confidence is normal.
- Attitude of self-identity.

CHARACTERISTICS OF MENTALLY HEALTHY PERSON

- A mentally healthy person is capable of solving his problems for adjustment.
- The mentally healthy person knows the priority of values and clarification in it. In failure of solutions, he tries to change his thoughts in a meaningful way. He is good in social interactions and fellow members.
- The mentally healthy person will be wise by showing efforts necessary in managing confidential issues toward his personal and social life.
- He gives priority by love and affection toward family by managing healthy relations, economic matters, etc.
- The mentally healthy person is emotionally matured, tolerates frustration by failures, and modifies his behavior toward success in it.

Physical health and mental health both are essential to lead healthy life. The modern concept of health is managing both physical and psychological well-being. The coordination of body and mind depends on healthy personal feelings, thoughts, controlling emotions, fulfilling desires, and ability to face and accept reality in development of personality.

WARNING SIGNS OF POOR MENTAL HEALTH

The person may lose temperament and shows anger for simple reasons.

The person with poor mental health is not interested in social relations, needs isolation, not punctual in working, and not bothered about personal life and responsibilities **(Fig. 7.2)**.

They maintain irregular and abnormal physiological conditions (blood pressure, heart palpitation, and pulse rate).

The above may cause threat to mental health. Sometimes it leads to criminal attitudes in fulfilling his sexual attitudes and even attempt of suicides.

The American Psychological Association, with help from First Lady Michelle Obama, has launched a campaign to encourage troubled Americans to seek care for mental health problems.

In addition, this initiative seeks to end the stigma associated with mental health issues. The campaign urges people to watch for five signs that someone is suffering from and may need help. They are:

1. **Changes in personality:** Someone who behaves as a different person without self-feeling, is one of the warning signs of poor mental health.
2. **Anxiety, anger, and moodiness:** Frequency of emotional changes is also an alarming symptom of poor mental health.
3. **Social withdrawal and isolation:** The poor mental health person is not interested in social relations and wants to be alone.
4. **Lack of Self-care or risky behavior:** The mentally poor health makes him to neglect his health, and the person mainly focuses on temporary relief by taking of alcohol and drugs.
5. **A sense of hopelessness:** These people may develop pessimistic attitudes, losing confidence to become normal.

They will get help of licensed, professional counselor or by support of local mental health association.

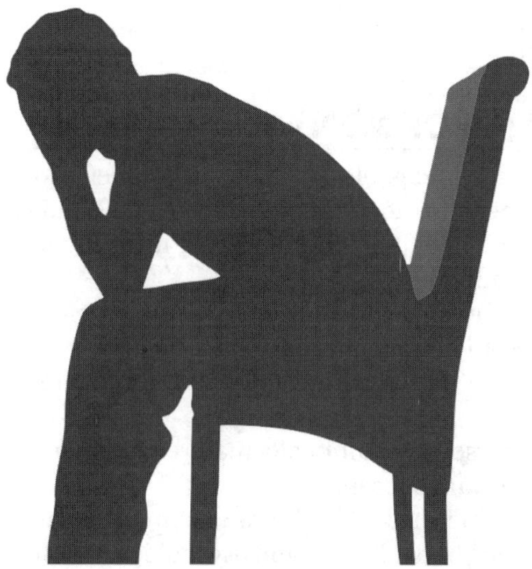

Fig. 7.2: Person suffering with mental illness

PROMOTION OF MENTAL HEALTH: STRATEGIES AND SERVICES

Promotion of mental health emphasized that early intervention and prevention are necessary.

The good mental health depends on healthy physical and social environment of human beings.

The development of personality begins from infant stage of life. The factors of healthy development of personality are attributed to heredity and environment. Parental care, love, and affection help in promotion of good mental health. A sound mental health can get altered due to inability to cope stress and conflicts, lack of rest and sleep, insufficient food, and lack of psychological support from family members. The most common mental illnesses in children include anxiety disorder, as well as depression in older children and teens.

Most of the adolescents face psychological trauma by maladjustment, gender differences, external pressures of education of teachers, parents, peer group, economic crisis, sexual feelings to opposite sex, etc.

Friends and families are having a major role in stabilizing and treating child's mental health.

PREVENTION

The early prevention is better than cure. Negligence of family, ill treatment, step parents, and broken families are main causes of mental ill-health. The care is essential from mother's womb which begins by intake of nutritious food, adapting coping strategies of stress in pregnancy, and timely infant care.

It is also necessary to consult the psychiatrist to avoid severity in later stages.

Prevention is beginning to appear in mental health strategies, including the 2004 WHO report "Prevention of Mental Disorders", the 2008 EU "Pact for Mental Health", and the 2011 US National Prevention Strategy. Prevention of a disorder at a young age may significantly decrease the chances that a child will suffer from a disorder later in life, and shall be the most efficient and effective measure from a public health perspective.

The new Mental Healthcare Bill that decriminalizes attempt to suicide and bans use of electric shock therapy for treating children with mental illness was passed by the Lok-Sabha on 10th April 1917 by the Indian Government. An estimated 6–7% of the country's population suffers from some kind of mental illness, while 1–2% has an acute condition.

Mental illness can be prevented in adults by providing healthy atmosphere of employment facilities, good family living, psychological support of family and friends, and social interactions.

In prevention of mental ill health, women need freedom in selection of life partner. They need psychological support from parents and social agencies to get higher education, to avoid dowry deaths and motivate self-confidence reduces mental tension in women.

Another way to improve our mental health is participating in activities of family get-together, touring, and spending time with loved ones.

Most of the people working in army and military are also facing problems in their working areas.

Special attention is also given to the adolescent students to tolerate distress by managing classes of Yoga, meditation, and other relaxation techniques, games, and sports.

Music Therapy

Activity therapies of dance, music, and other recreational activities are other stress coping techniques. These are called as expressive therapies.

Did you know?

In 1919, Maharaja of Vijay Nagar kingdom Pusapati Vijyarama Gajapathi Raju's assistant was not happy due to the blindness of his son. He loved music. In that situation, their family expressed to king about the cause of depression of his son. The king bought veena (music instrument) for assistant's son. The king supported and established one music college near his Mahal. It was developed as Sri Vijayarama Music and Dance College.

Later the blind became a popular "violin musician" (**Fig. 7.3**).

Most of the Andhra Pradesh singers learn music in that college. Nearly 7,000 musicians have learned music in that college.

Most of these therapies of dance and music are more popular in modern days for the recovery of mental disorders.

Group Therapy

In group therapy, different cases come into light for treatment. In these therapies, people get more benefits compared to individual treatment. People openly discuss their problems toward treatment of the complaint. The other members of the group may get confidence and emotionally cooperate in description of their problems. The group is effective in changing the thinking, attitude, and feelings of group members.

Group therapy is also being implemented in treating addiction of alcohol and other substance use. It takes place with a group of people together rather than with an individual during a one-on-one session. It is a psychological therapy in treatment of addiction. It can reduce the anxiety levels of mentally ill.

Schizophrenia: It is a psychological disorder. Group therapy for those with schizophrenia can be beneficial, depending on the severity of the condition. It can be helpful to reach out to others who experience similar symptoms in group and learning more about the disorder can help to understand own thoughts better.

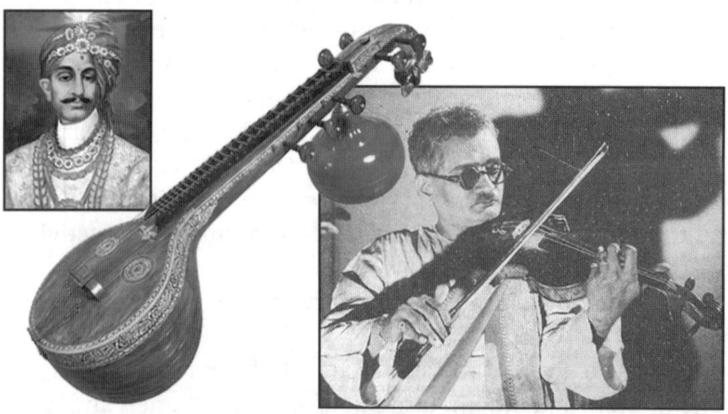

Fig. 7.3: The blind person became a famous musician

Psychotherapy

Psychotherapy is the general term for scientific based treatment of mental health issues based on modern medicine. Majority of psycho-education is provided to healthy living. These are motivating techniques in school children, especially adolescents, to avoid self-harm and to balance stress. It is helping for behavior modification in adolescents to create interest in life skills and mindfulness.

Meditation

The management of good mental health is followed by relaxation technique of meditation **(Fig. 7.4)**. It is followed since our ancestral days. In modern days also, most of people do meditation. It reduces anxiety, depression, and frustrations. It brings some changes in brain and circulation of blood.

Spiritual Counseling

Spiritual counselors meet with people to offer comfort and support and to help them gain a better understanding of their issues and develop a problem-solving relation with spirituality. These types of counselors deliver care based on spiritual, psychological, and theological principles.

The people who believe in spirituality give priority to yoga and meditation as relaxation techniques to promote mental health. Indian Prime Minister Narendra Modi said "lifestyle and stress-related diseases are becoming more and more common today. The whole world wants peace...not only from war and conflict but peace of mind," he said, adding Yoga was the "sharpest weapon" to beat stress.

Social work in mental health: The relation between mental health and social work is an old process. Some people enjoy doing service to the public and may get peace to their mind. The different religious groups in many countries believe that serving to people is equal to prayer of God. Social workers provide individual home visits for mentally ill and do welfare services; with specialized training, a range of procedural services are coordinated for home, workplace,

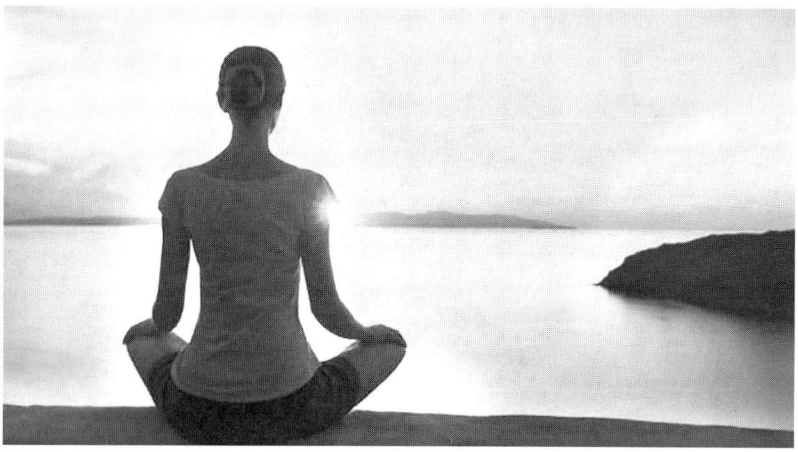

Fig. 7.4: Meditation as relaxation technique

and school. Social workers play many roles in mental health settings, including those of case manager, advocate, administrator, and therapist. Social work is a professional degree in mental health called as psychiatric social work. Psychiatric social workers are mental health professionals that can assist patients and their family members in coping with both mental health issues and various economic or social problems caused by mental illness. Psychiatric social workers who provide assessment and psychosocial interventions function in clinical side, counselors are working in communities and the health centers. The major functions of a psychiatric social worker are promotion and prevention, treatment, and rehabilitation.

Many nongovernmental organizations (NGO) are doing services for the well-being of mentally ill. In the United States, social workers provide most of the mental health services. According to government sources, 60% of mental health professionals are clinically trained social workers, compared to 10% of psychiatrists, 23% of psychologists, and 5% of psychiatric nurses.

INDIA—MENTAL HEALTH FACILITIES

In Mughal period, Unani system of medicine was introduced by Indian physician Unhammad in 1922. In 1745, lunatic asylums were started in Mumbai followed by Calcutta in 1784, and Chennai in 1794. The first lunatic act came into effect in India in 1912.

A rehabilitation program was initiated and Mysore Lunatic Asylum was started in 1847; and the department was established for occupational therapy. This was the beginning of psychosocial education in India.

In 1937, the first post of psychiatric social worker was created in the child guidance clinic run by the Dhorabji Tata School of Social Work (established in 1936). It is considered as the first documented evidence of social work practice in Indian mental health field.

In1960, at the All India Institute of Medical Sciences in Delhi, and in 1960, the Madras Mental Hospital (Now Institute of Mental Health), employed social workers to bridge the gap between doctors and patients.

In 1847, Bangalore Lunatic Asylum was founded by Dr Charles Irwing Smith, a British medical practitioner in Bangalore. In 1961, the social work post was created at the NIMHANS (National Institute of Mental Health and Neuro Sciences), Bangalore **(Fig. 7.5)**.

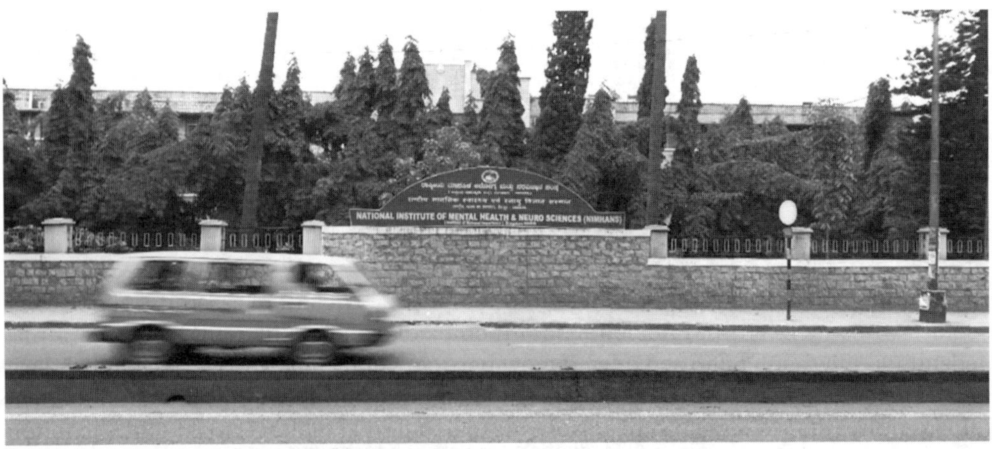

Fig. 7.5: Mental hospital, NIMHANS, Bangalore

A new initiative to integrate mental health with general health services started in 1975 in India. The Ministry of Health, Government of India, formulated the National Mental Health Programme (NMHP) and launched it in 1982. The same was reviewed in 1995 and based on that, the District Mental Health Programme (DMHP) was launched in 1996 and sought to integrate mental healthcare with public healthcare. This model has been implemented in all the states and currently there are 125 DMHP sites in India.

National Human Rights Commission (NHRC) in 1998 and 2008 carried out systematic, intensive, and critical examinations of mental hospitals in India.

In 2016, Mental Health Care Bill was passed which ensures and legally entitles access to treatments with coverage from insurance, safeguarding dignity of the afflicted person, improving healthcare access, and free medications.

EGO DEFENSE MECHANISMS

Ego defense mechanisms are called as adjustment mechanisms and mental mechanisms. The satisfaction of ego is not a difficult task. It stands on reality principle. Sometimes, it creates tensions in human mind. The protection of these trends in healthy way is called defense mechanisms.

Definition

Defense mechanism is a process in the brain that makes us forget or ignore painful or disturbing thoughts and situations.

A reaction in our body that protects against disease or danger.

Medical definition of defense mechanism as often unconscious mental process (as repression, projection, or sublimation).

Bhatia and Craig: "The individual has mental capacities or devices for protecting himself against psychological dangers and distress."

The defense mechanisms are unconscious behavioral patterns. The concept of defense mechanism was proposed by Sigmund Freud in 1904 by applying to the unconscious process. The suppression of unpleasant impulses of anxiety will be progress until the conflict is resolved.

Types of Defense Mechanisms (Fig. 7.6)

Projection

In a way it is a form of rationalization, because it excuses failure and places faults on others. Different age people use these in different levels of their life. Some people cannot tolerate failures and instead of accepting them as their mistakes they are ready to throw blame on others. This method is very common. Projection is often the result of a lack of insight and acknowledgement of one's own motivations and feelings.

Sublimation

Sublimation is simply the channeling of unacceptable drive or urge into a form that is acceptable to society. In fulfilling the desires, some thoughts are harmful. To suppress these feelings, diversion is very important. The process in which an individual chooses another process to divert his mind is called sublimation, e.g., sexual thoughts. In country like India, values and

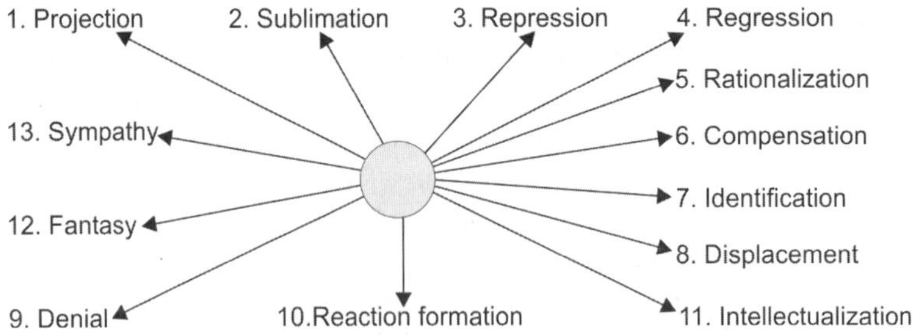

Fig. 7.6: List of defense mechanisms

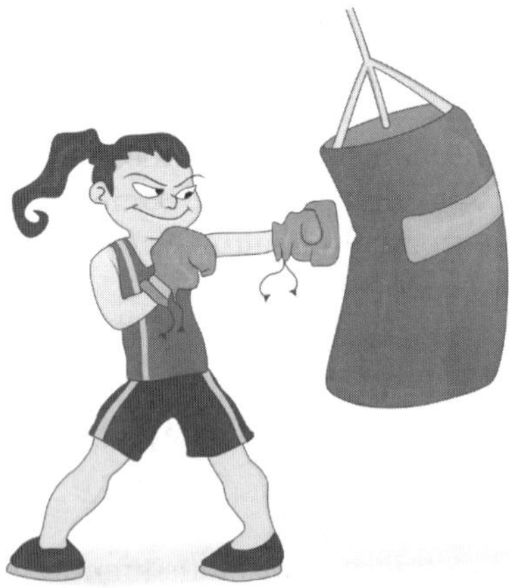

- Channeling of unacceptable and potentially disruptive impulses, thoughts or emotions into socially acceptable behavior.
- Dealing with emotional stressors by using the energy in other, usually constructive activities.
- Ex: Punching bag to channel angry impulses. Sports.

Fig. 7.7: Sublimation of defense mechanism

culture are more important to marriage and family. The harmful thoughts create danger to both personal and social life.

Sublimation can also be done with humor or fantasy **(Fig. 7.7)**. Humor reduces the intensity of a situation, and places a cushion of laughter between the person and the impulses.

Repression

Repression is one of the defense mechanisms to forcefully suppress our painful thoughts and anxiety-based feelings in unconscious level. It makes us behave normally in day-to-day life. This way of suppressing is called repression. Preventing painful or dangerous thoughts from entering consciousness is known as reaction formation.

A conscious perception of instincts and feelings is blocked in repression.

Regression

Regression is a process of unconscious forgetfulness and conflict-producing emotions and desires. It occurs when, in response to some threat, a person returns to an earlier stage of development. For example, the young married woman who has difficulties with her husband may plan to spend time with her parents. Some regressions such as tears, become more emotional while facing problems in life. Extreme forms and degree of repression result in psychosis.

Rationalization

In this type of defense mechanism, the individual justifies his failures and anti-social behavior by socially acceptable reasons. For example, an employee who loses his job expresses that in another way of insufficient salary or improper management, etc. A student who fails in examination may convey that teachers are not good in his school.

In rationalization, the person wants to cover his mistakes by throwing blame on others; sour grapes (Fox and Grape story) and sweet lemon etc.

Compensation

Many people use compensation to enhance their self-esteem and prestige. It refers to more or less unconsciously motivated behavior whose purpose is to make up for what the individual feels what he lost. The student not be interested to continue his education and shows interest in games and sports. Many eminent persons have done remarkable things in life just to compensate for what they lacked in other directions.

Identification

In this defense mechanism, the individual feels personal satisfaction in success and achievement by competing with others in groups. Most of the children in family want to identify themselves; girl imitates their mother and boy imitates their father. Youngsters will identify themselves as hero or heroine while watching movies. They identify every successful and healthy way to develop their attitudes. It is a healthy development by imagining valuable future.

Displacement

Displacement is the redirecting of thoughts, feelings, and impulses focused at one person or object taken to another person **(Fig. 7.8)**. The people who avoid their feelings of anger, fear, etc., react on children and pet animals to suppress their feeling. In this way, they will satisfy their feelings and become normal.

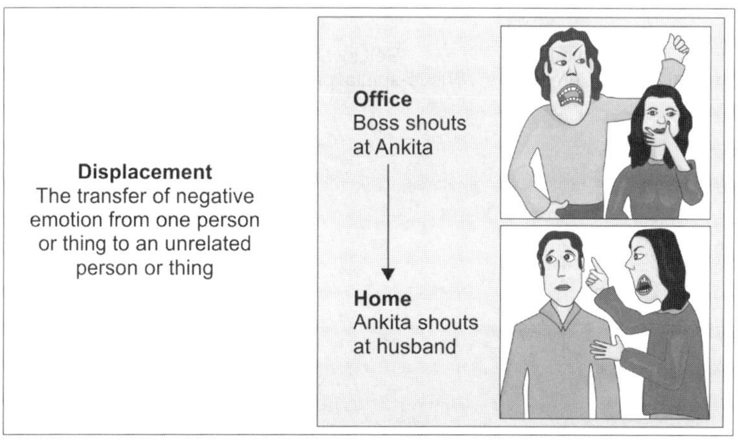

Fig. 7.8: Displacement of defense mechanism

Denial

Denial is planned ordinary rejection. It is a method of resolving conflict that all persons use to extent. In denial, the individual does not accept the existence of something that is disturbing. In fact, the denial of illness is a fairly common behavior pattern in medical settings.

Reaction Formation

It is a conversion from dangerous feelings to secured techniques. A job holder who is very angry with his boss would like to quit his job instead of accepting their boss with politeness. He is not capable of expressing his anger and unhappiness on boss.

Intellectualization

Intellectualization is a form of isolation, concentrating the intellectual components of a situation so as to distance oneself from the associated anxiety-provoking emotions, separation of emotion from ideas, thinking about wishes in formal, affectively mild terms and not acting on them, avoiding unacceptable emotions by focusing on the intellectual aspects. For instance, a person who has just been given a terminal medical diagnosis, instead of expressing his sadness and grief, focuses on the details of all possible fruitless medical procedures.

Fantasy or Daydreaming

Fantasy is also a kind of withdrawal when facing real problems of life. Daydreaming helps in making adjustment. Gratifying frustrated desires by imaginary achievements is called fantasy. Most of the youth imagines their life with beautiful dreams, luxurious life, successful desires, and relaxing from pressures and pains of present situations. Its extreme is also very dangerous to their mental health and long duration of daydreaming leads to psychotic disorder called schizophrenia. It is not possible to realize truth and present situation of their life.

Sympathy

Sympathy: It is defense mechanism in which a person invites sympathy in a difficult situation **(Fig. 7.9)**.

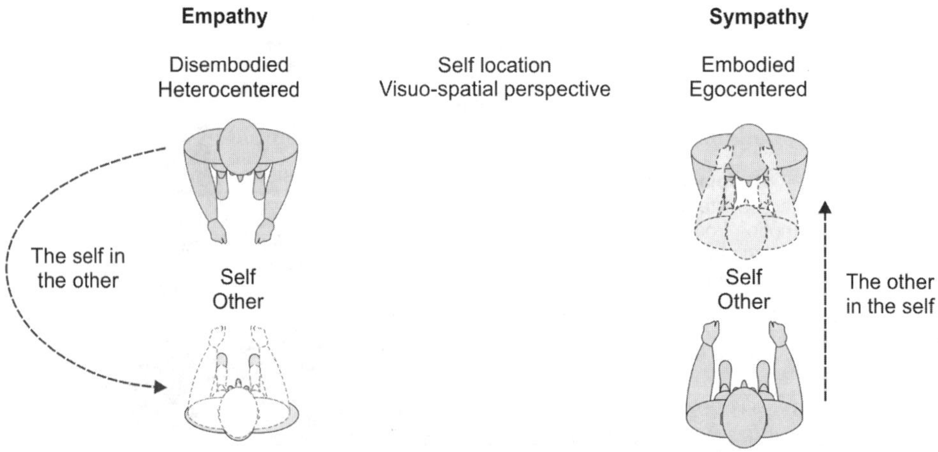

Fig. 7.9: Sympathy as defense mechanism

Empathy: Empathy is the ability to share another person's feelings and emotions as if they were your own. It is the projection of one's own personality into the personality of another in order to understand the person better, ability to share other's emotions, thoughts, or feelings.

PERSONAL AND SOCIAL ADJUSTMENT

In modern society, psychology is helping in adjustment—both personal and social adjustment. Psychological perspectives and concepts are focusing on coping stress, toleration of frustrations by using some relaxation techniques, to control highly emotional attitudes in personality, and social adjustment. In primary stages of maladjustment, it can be treated by counseling strategies, hypnotism, and body relaxation techniques; yoga and meditation are more helpful in prevention of mental illness as psychotherapy.

Social competence, like social adjustment, is often used as an umbrella term to include various aspects of a child's performance in social contexts. Those who design and provide programs for preschoolers and school-aged children in group settings often seek to enhance aspects of personal and social adjustment, either as a primary outcome or as a valued by-product of other program activities (Hauser-Cram and Shonkoff, 1988; Ysseldyke and Thurlow, 1993).

Every individual is born in a society which influences our behavior by social situations like family, education, working environment, and community. Their influence has major role on our mental status.

On occasion of World Heart Day, 2017, Dr B Soma Raju, a famous cardiologist from Hyderabad, explained that family and society both are having major role on healthy life of the individual and group **(Fig. 7.10)**.

Broken families, step parents, ill-treatment in the family, financial sources, unemployment, drought situations, natural calamities, and war are some other reasons for social maladjustment.

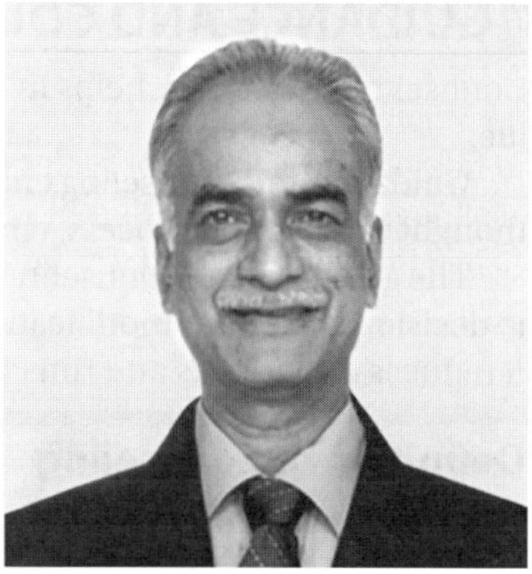

Fig. 7.10: Dr B Soma Raju Cardiologist Padma Sree Award by Government of India 2001

The medical team is doing research to motivate healthy behavior in treating physical sickness. The Government is planning to recruit psychologists in work-places on personality development programs to avoid frustrations and even suicidal tendencies among the people. It helps them face the failures or loss in their personal and social life.

The articles connected to social adjustment are getting more prominence by usage of mobile messages and newspapers by experts of psychological field. It is creating emotional and cognitive skills to manage relations in healthy way.

Extracurricular activities such as games, sports, and competitions promote the physical and emotional development in school children. In modern days, schools are encouraging children toward Yoga and meditation to feel free from distress.

The draught and cyclones and other natural calamities make the villagers feel distress.

The distress in farmers is also giving chance for suicidal deaths, addiction of drugs, and other substance use.

The encouragement of group activities, e.g., "Mela" as some recreational activities **(Fig. 7.11)**, leads to good social relations among villagers.

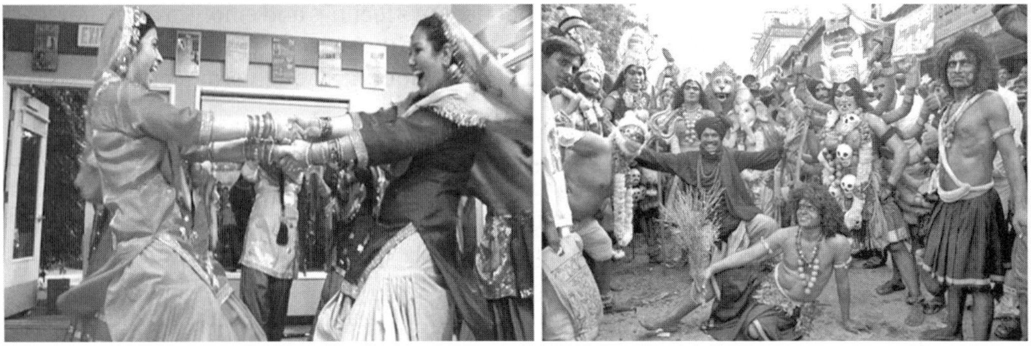

Fig. 7.11: Recreation by Mela's for managing social relation

According to Sigmund Freud, the primary level experiences up to the age of 5 years have more influence on their future behavior of individuals. The foundation of basics is very strong toward the behavior future, social interactions, emotional attitudes of short temper, aggressive behavior, and toleration of success and failures in concept of Freud. But it is not giving clarity on influence of the behavior of humans and dependence of primary level experiences. The care and responsibility, relationship among family members, teachers' care, and community influence the children to learn good manners and help them in personal and social adjustments. It provides self-confidence to lead independent life and decision-making abilities toward their future life. This is another factor in the development of sound mental health.

GUIDANCE AND COUNSELING

Counseling psychology helps in safeguarding the future problems of both personal and social life.

Guidance and counseling enable the individual to understand his or her abilities, interests, thought content and process, emotions, motives, conflicts, etc.

The guidance and counseling make the individual to think his own problems and strategies in decision-making by modification of behavior to compromise on several issues by analyzation. It reduces day dreams and runs to real world by capability of skills.

Definition of Counseling

The term counseling is relationship in which one person endeavors to help another to understand and solve his adjustment problems—**English and english dictionary**.

"Counseling is face-to-face relationship in which growth takes place in the counselor as well as the counselee"—**Ruth Strang**.

Counseling means the client to express his or her feelings with counselor and discuss the problems to safeguard his or her life. These are confidential because these are client's personal matters. It is not a single-day process.

Counseling is a profession by a qualified psychologist. The advices and judgment are very important in identification of problem and solution to proceed to counsel and provide confidence to the client to tell the truth without hesitation. It depends on talent of counselor in rapport with client. Relationship between counselor and counselee is characterized by trust, warmth, and understanding.

Types of Counseling

- Psychological counseling
- Psycho-therapeutic counseling
- Student counseling
- Marriage counseling
- Vocational counseling
- Motivational counseling
- Group counseling

In general, the feelings of happy, sad, and angry emotions are common in individual behavior.

The counseling psychology focuses on treating individuals with a variety of emotional, behavioral, and social problems or disorders. Clinical psychologists and counseling psychologists both deal with wide variety of mental and emotional problems. Counseling psychologists typically focus on individuals whose symptoms are less severe, such as those coping with stress and adjusting to life. Clinical psychologists, on the other hand, treat patients with more serious symptoms and disorders.

Sigmund Freud opened his private practice in 1886 and treated his patients with counseling and therapy.

Lightner Witmer opened one of the first psychological clinics, a short time later, in 1896.

Carl Rogers was also one of the founding fathers of person-centered therapy, which is a type of therapy that is based on the patient's own individual life experiences.

Cognitive behavioral therapy is another common type of treatment used by cognitive psychologists.

The majority of counseling psychologists interact with their patients each and every day. They are often presented with a wide range of mental and emotional problems that people face every day.

Guidance and Counseling

This process is helping individuals in coping in educational, vocational, and psychological problems. It is a therapy to achieve happy and adjustable status from complicated situations. The person who faces mental strain will approach these professionals.

"Guidance is a process of helping every individual through his own efforts to discover and develop his potentialities for his personal happiness and social usefulness."—**Ruth Strang**

Guidance, in this sense, is a pervasive activity in which many persons and organizations take part. Some of the government and non-government organizations take the support of family counselors to tackle issues between marital couples, e.g., domestic violence, problem by giving birth to a girl child, harassment by in-laws, etc.

Guidance is an educational service designed to help students to make more effective use of the school's training program. Professional counselors and counseling psychologists are commonly found in institutional settings such as high schools and colleges, private industry, community agencies, prisons, and the military, as well as in private practice.

Differences between Guidance versus Counseling

	Guidance	*Counseling*
1.	Guidance is to provide solution to focused problems by qualified experts	Counseling is advice from a professional counselor to overcome psychological problems
2.	Guidance is an external analysis of problem	Counseling is an internal analysis of the problem
3.	Guidance supports in decision-making	Counseling is a remedial process for healthy living
4.	Guidance is an awareness of personal problems like education	Counseling is on personal and social issues
5.	Guidance is to develop self-direction to improve the skills in solving problems	Counseling is a helping service. It helps the individual to help himself
6.	Guidance is a process to help individual in searching of resources to solve his problems	Counseling is a psychotherapy to help the suffering from mild mental disorders
7.	Guidance is based on generalized and specialized services	Counseling emphasizes on social, personal, and emotional problem

CONCLUSION

The knowledge on mental health and mental hygiene helps nurse. The treatment is appreciated by the recovery of patient to normal status. It is also gaining support of family members in guiding them to create peaceful atmosphere, not to repeat the complicated situation in family, and social adjustment.

QUESTIONS

Essay Questions

1. Define guidance and counseling. List down the principles of guidance and counseling.
2. Define defense mechanism and explain any five defense mechanisms with examples.

Short Notes

1. Write briefly on warning signs of poor mental health.
2. Define sublimation.
3. Characteristics of mentally healthy person.
4. Explain the role of nurse in counseling.
5. List down the principles of counseling.
6. What are the steps to prevent mental and emotional disturbances?
7. Guidance and counseling.
8. Explain any two defense mechanisms with examples.
9. Explain the promotive mental health strategies and services.

Brief Questions

1. Define defense mechanism.
2. Enumerate any two warning signs of poor mental health.

3. Mental hygiene.
4. Personal and social adjustment in mental hygiene.
5. Define guidance.
6. Differentiate between projection and rationalization.

Fill in the Blanks

1. WHO definition of ______________ "A state of complete physical, mental, and social well-being and not merely the absence of disease or infirmity". (health)
2. Schizophrenia is ______________ disorder. (psychological)
3. ______________ is a process in the brain that makes us to forget or ignore painful or disturbing thoughts and situations. (Defense mechanism)
4. ______________ is an educational service designed to help students to make more effective use of the school's training programs. (Guidance)
5. Gratifying frustrated desires by imaginary achievements is called ______________ (fantasy).
6. Preventing painful or dangerous thoughts from entering conscious is known as ______________ (repression).
7. ______________ is the ability to share another person's feelings and emotions as if they were your own. (Empathy)

Multiple Choice Questions

1. Ego defence mechanisms ....
   a. Guidance
   b. Repression
   c. Counseling
2. .... is an educational service designed to help students make more effective use the school's training program.
   a. Guidance
   b. Denial
   c. Displacement
3. Fantasy or daydreaming is one of the ....
   a. Mental health
   b. Counseling
   c. Defence mechanisms

Answers

1. b	2. a	3. c

8 CHAPTER

Psychological Assessment and Tests

Learning Objectives

- Psychological assessment and tests
- Types, development, characteristics, principles, uses, interpretation, and role of nurse in psychological assessment

PSYCHOLOGICAL TESTS AND ASSESSMENTS

The roots of psychological testing were traced back to centuries. The ancient Greeks applied testing in a systematic way to assess both physical and mental powers. In the recent years, experimental psychologists like Cattell, Galton, Pearson, and Binet contributed remarkably for the growth, development, and evaluation of psychological tests.

Psychological test and assessment is the foundation in judging the psychological behavior of individual or groups. Technical term for psychological testing is psychometrics.

Psychological testing may be defined as a process of forming an overall impression on judgment about the person regarding his behavior, personality traits, nature of adjustment, achievements and abilities, moods and motivations, goals and aspirations, etc.

Psychological testing uses some tools in diagnosing for treatment. It is administered in both children and adults differentiated by their age. In adults, these are useful in measuring the occupational skills. These are standardized in assessment of objectivity in decision-making toward particular skill of employment. These are done by qualified experts to diagnose slow learners, loss of memory, etc. In psychological assessment, the expert is also interested to know the genetic disorders or brain injuries for changes in mental health.

In psychological assessment, personal interaction with client is more useful in observing the facial feelings and changing levels in emotional attitudes of interaction. The psychological assessments may also include interviewing other people who are close to the client, such as teachers, co-workers, or family members. Sometimes the written information and ability of writing skills are used to assess intelligence of the client. It gives clarity on assessment of psychological levels of the individual by comparison of their physical age. Psychological assessment is concerned mainly by empirical research on measurement and evaluation of psychological problems done by psychiatrist or clinical psychologist.

Both testing and assessment allow a psychologist to see the full picture of a person's strengths and limitations. These are like medical tests, in observing the X-ray and blood tests to develop the treatment plans of physical ill-health. Psychological symptoms are not stable in the patient. Sometimes the test results are not possible to cover all psychological symptoms accurately, so it causes difficulty in diagnoses of mental illness. Psychological assessment is performed in formal manner only by a qualified and expert in subject. Psychologists use tests and other assessment tools to measure and observe a client's behavior in diagnosis and to guide in treatment. So the analytical team uses different techniques in diagnosing. Psychologists administer tests and assessments in a wide variety of reasons. Children who are experiencing difficulty in school, for example, may undergo aptitude tests to know learning disabilities. Tests in skills such as dexterity, reaction time, and memory can help a neuropsychologist to diagnose the conditions such as brain injuries or dementia.

PSYCHOLOGICAL TESTS

Psychological tests are classified in several ways **(Fig. 8.1):**

1. Individual vs. group tests
2. Paper vs. performance test
3. Verbal vs. nonverbal tests
4. Speed vs. power tests
5. Formal and informal tests.

Ability Tests

Aptitude Tests

Aptitude is a special skill of measuring intelligence levels in different interests of music, art, mechanism, religious views, etc.

Aptitude assessment is used to predict success or failures in activity. These are used to test vocational skills, career guidance in assessment of numerical ability, learning ability, verbal ability, and clerical perception.

Examples—Minnesota mechanical assessment test
Scholastic aptitude test (SAT)
Differentiate aptitude test (DAT).

Psychological tests measure specific abilities, such as clerical, perceptual, numerical, or spatial aptitude (SAT).

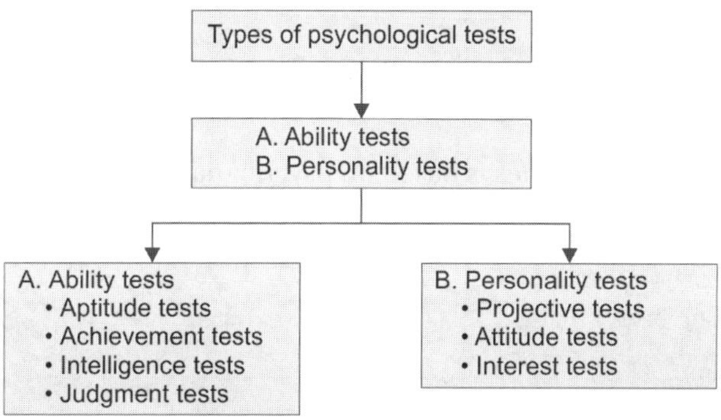

Fig. 8.1: Types of psychological tests

Achievement Tests

Achievement tests are used in assessing a person what he achieved, acquired, or learnt.

Example of achievement test: Wechsler Individual Achievement Test (WIAT).

Intelligence Tests

1. Stanford-Binet test
2. Wechsler Adult Intelligence Scale (WAIS)
3. Raven's Progressive Matrices (RPM).

Intelligence tests are used to measure a person's overall level of intellectual functioning. Intelligence tests are used in assessing the intelligence or level of cognitive functioning of the individual.

The Stanford-Binet Intelligence Scale is a popular intelligence test. It can be administered from age 2 through late adulthood.

Wechsler Adult Intelligence Scale (WAIS)

The Wechsler Intelligence Scale for Children-III (WISC-III).

Judgment Tests

Situational judgment tests were mostly used in World War II by the psychologists in US.

Today, SJTs are used in many organizations and are promoted by various consulting firms.

Personality Tests

Personality tests are self-reported inventories that are used to assess personal traits and behaviors. Some of these tests also cover much information on health-related issues of substance abuse, anxiety, depression, and other psychological symptoms.

Minnesota Multiphasic Personality Inventory (MMPI)
Sixteen Personality Factor Questionnaire (16 PF)
Eysenck Personality Inventory
Rorschach Inkblot Test (RIT)
Thematic Apperception Test (TAT)
Observational techniques, Questionnaire
Interview
Rating scales.

Projective Techniques

The aim of the projective techniques is based on psychoanalysis.

Rorschach Ink Blot Test
TAT-Thematic Apperception Test
Children's Apperception Test
Word Association Test
Sentence Completion Test
Picture Arrangement Test.

Attitude Test

Attitude test assesses an individual's feelings and behavior. Attitude scale is used to train in sales and marketing to convince the minds toward purchase of items. Example—Thurston Scale of Likert Scale.

Semantic Differential (SD) is another type of attitude test for rating.

Interest Tests

Interest tests are depending on personal priority of education and employment sectors. A widely used interest test is the Strong Interest Inventory which is used in career counseling and educational guidance.

DEVELOPMENT OF PSYCHOLOGICAL TESTING (FIG. 8.2)

In psychological assessment, psychological tests are aptitude tests, achievement test used for occupation, counseling, management skills, and career planning.

Clinical Interview

Psychological tests are used in clinical setting to diagnose treatment. Professionals are serious in gathering information by different tests of observation. Clinical interview is a component in psychological setting.

Intelligence Assessment

Intelligence tests are helpful in understanding learning disorders, measuring the mental disorders, and improving abilities and motivational skills by performance tasks, e.g. verbal and nonverbal test, language skills, word association or sentence completion tests, solving puzzles, symbols, etc.

Career Development

Aptitude tests to know the special abilities, interest toward particular job, in development of business, achievement tests of task performance, projective techniques in job recruitment, career counseling are helpful in development of psychological tests. In school children, these tests usually include development of sensory and motor skills, language skills, and simple cognitive skills.

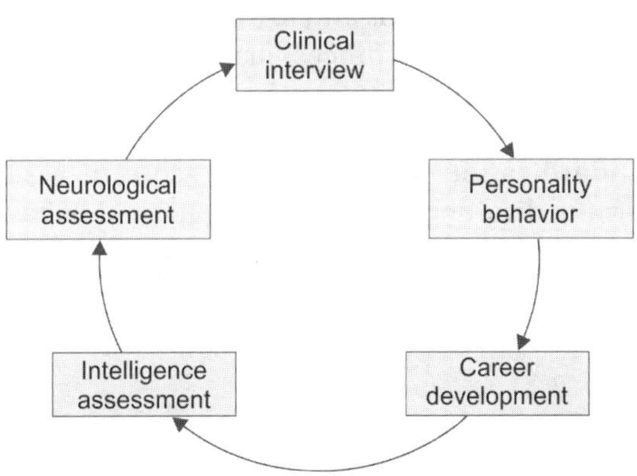

Fig. 8.2: Development of psychological testing

Neuropsychological Assessment

Neuropsychological tests are used in assessment of persons with known or suspected malfunctioning of brain. Neuropsychology is the study of brain-behavior relationships.

Neuropsychological tests consist of specifically designed tasks used to measure a psychological function known to be linked to a particular brain structure or pathway. The collected data of neurological test help in assessment of psychological disorders, defects of neurological function, impairment, brain injuries, etc.

Intelligence tests are helpful to know the neuropsychological problems. Common types administered include the Stanford-Binet and the Wechsler scales. Advanced radiological techniques such as computerized tomography (CT) and magnetic resonance imaging (MRI) are used to know the causes of brain damage.

Personality Behavior

Psychological measures of personality are often described as either objective tests or projective tests. The rating scales, self-reporting tests, attitude, and interest help in development of psychological testing. Objective observation of cognitive behavior provides information about adaptive and maladaptive aspects of people's thoughts and the role their thoughts play in the processes of planning and making decisions.

CHARACTERISTICS OF PSYCHOLOGICAL TESTING

Sample of Behavior

It motivates rest of the information for stabilization. The term of sample of behavior is possible individual task performance in different verbal and non-verbal tests, interview, observation, and intelligence tests. Sample of behavior is the characteristic of psychological tests.

Standardization

Standardized testing procedure is an essential feature of psychological test. A psychological test is a sample of behavior collected under standardized conditions. The standard is not simple process; it is fixed by different samples, proofs of observation in psychological test. It refers to the consistency of the conditions and in systematic procedure for administering a test. The vague information is difficult in process of diagnosis for treatment of psychological symptoms of the patient. A large diversity exists among different psychological tests and thousands of different tests in the market. The continuation of development of psychological tests depends on standardization. The results of score in assessment are useful in improvement from learning disorders and in modification of behavior. Differences in test scores are thought to reflect individual differences in the construct the test is supposed to measure.

Psychometrics

The technical term for the science behind psychological testing is psychometrics. In psychometric test, items will be ordered in level of difficulty, so that the candidate can solve test easily; weaker candidate cannot face complex items early.

"Psychometric" is a term coined by Joseph R. It is psychological ability of sensation of touch and assesses the values. Examples are sound, smell, taste, vision, color, etc. The levels of emotions formed by sensations. The psychic may not be able to do this with all objects at all times and, as with all psychic abilities, accuracy can vary, but the ability is available to the psychic.

Norms

Psychometric tests and questionnaires are usually scored objectively. Scores on psychological tests rarely provide absolute ratio scale measure of psychological attributes, intelligence, motivation, depth perception, and so on. A norm-based score indicates where an individual stands in comparison to the particular normative group that defines the set of standards. One of the most useful ways of describing a person's performance on a test is to compare his or her test score to the scores of some other person or group of people.

Reliability

The fundamental purpose of standardizing a psychological test is to establish its reliability and validity. Reliability and validity are two essential characteristics. A test is reliable to the extent that it measures whatever is measured consistently. In testing a coefficient of reliability, errors of measurement have been reduced to minimum. Reliable tests are stable. Reliability is the self-consistence of test. A reliable test need not always be valid but a valid test is always reliable.

Validity

The type of test being administered must measure what it is intended to measure. It is also thought of utility. There are different types of validity tests, like content validity, especially importance of achievement is very much important in aptitude tests. The testing tools give information in both reliability and validity of test in its manual. Validity test indicates the truth.

THE PRINCIPLES OF PSYCHOLOGICAL ASSESSMENT

The psychological test is based on procedure. It makes possible for administration. The sample behavior interest permits the administrator to make inference about the domain of relevant behavior.

A psychological test must also permit the derivation of scores or categories. Every test furnishes one or more scores or provides evidence that a person belongs to one category. The scores earned by an individual on a psychological test should be properly interpreted on the basis of norms laid down in the test manual for providing clear direction where the individual stands in comparison to others in the matter of possession of the measured psychological attribute.

The purpose of testing is to estimate the amount of the trait or characteristic being measured in different processes.

The subject provides an overview and critical evaluation of various tests currently used within applied areas of psychology, with an emphasis on personality and cognitive assessment.

The main principles of psychological tests are based on standardization, sample behavior, objectivity, norms, reliability, and validity.

USES OF PSYCHOLOGICAL TESTS

The most common use of psychological test is to make decision about persons. These are useful in education setting, to determine placement levels for students in universities to ascertain who should be admitted, on basis of score, local and civil service system by tests for purpose of personal selection.

Psychologists primarily use tests to supplement or assist in various phases of treatment. Test results used along with clinical discussions help us to move from one phase of treatment to the next. Tests that measure symptoms provide a picture of what needs to be changed. Individual practitioner exploits test in decision-making. Neuropsychologist uses this to check the function of brain.

Some other significant uses are diagnosis, treatment, planning, self-knowledge, program evaluation, and research. It is helpful in clinical interview and in psychiatric diagnosis.

The tests are used in forensic evaluation, family court, or criminal charges.

Psychologists use test results to help us in setting goals for improvement. Psychologists use unusual results, such as a high occurrence of depression, to develop specific and measurable goals.

Determining Interventions

Psychologists also use tests to identify the most effective interventions for us. Personality tests, such as the Myers-Briggs Type Indicator, can reveal much about how we think and the way we relate to other people. These tests reveal our strengths as well as our weaknesses. For example, our test results reveal that we are a highly analytical person; interventions such as reading and rational analysis of problems may be effective in helping us in making desired changes.

Reviewing Progress

Most psychologists use tests as a way of reviewing what we have accomplished in treatment. If the score is high on the Beck Anxiety Inventory in the initial assessment, re-taking the test 3 months later may reveal lower anxiety and provide us with momentum to keep up the work.

Closure:

A psychologist does not want the client to depend on him in decision-making; he tries to manage the client to get confidence in getting solutions of the problems. Psychologists often use tests as a way of ending treatment. Tests results are used as evidence in closing discussions about the progress they have achieved.

NATURE AND USE OF PSYCHOLOGICAL TESTS

The function of psychological test is to measure the difference between individuals or between the reactions of the same individual under different circumstances.

The Binet Intelligence test is useful in identification of mentally retarded person by applying the psychological tests.

Assessment of education: Classification of children with reference to their ability (differentiation of instructions).

We can identify outstanding slow or fast learners, educational occupational counseling of high school and college students, and selection of applicants for professional schools.

Selection and classification of industrial personnel tests: In job assignment, transfer, promotion, or termination can be identified by these tests. Educational vocational plans to involve with all aspects of person's life; emotional well-being and effective interpersonal relation have become increasingly prominent objectives of counseling.

Self-understanding: These tests are useful in self-understanding and personal development within this framework; test scores are given as an idea to one's decision-making processes. These tests are also useful in precise measurement of individual differences by well-constructed tests on basic researches, providing standardized tools, investigations, and development changes.

The tests are helpful in assessing the administration, cognitive abilities, interpersonal behavior, attitudes, and values. Personality tests are administered for a wide variety of reasons from diagnosing psychopathology (e.g. personality disorder).

Psychological tests are formalized in measuring mental functions. Projective tests may involve some level of subjective interpretation also known as inventories, measurements, questionnaires, and scales. Psychological tests are administrated in a variety of settings including preschools, primary and secondary schools, colleges and universities, hospitals, outpatient, healthcare settings, and social agencies.

Tests and Test Interpretation: Evaluation of the benefit of psychological comprehension test.

The findings of this examination are presented in relation to—(1) test description, (2) purpose of the test and population target, (3) test norm population, (4) factors measured by the test, and (5) test strengths and weaknesses.

PROFESSIONAL PSYCHOLOGY

Different schools of psychology developed and included analytical, behavioral, and humanistic ways. Primary contributors to American psychology were often educated in conjunction with Wundt's laboratory in Germany; they pursued academic careers with traditional experimental psychology and later developed applied interests.

Due to the increase in testing, it is vital for educators, especially classroom teachers who are responsible for preparing the students for these tests, to be aware of the impact of test anxiety.

Behavioral assessment procedures and vocational testing are other areas found in community psychology. This area includes the use of many tests included in the Vocational Preference Inventory (VPI).

Applications of Personality Tests: Personality tests are used in a variety of psychological settings. Objective tests are structured and assess the personality with specific test items; this is useful when behavioral and other approaches are considered; both types of personality tests are useful depending on the goals of testing.

Psychological tests are used in detection of specific behavior.

A psychological test is used to measure the individual differences that are different between abilities of different persons and performance of the same person at different time.

Psychological tests are used to diagnose mental disorders. So these tests are used in mental hospitals, counseling, and guidance centers for the assessment of mental disorders.

A psychological test helps in classifying a number of people into different categories like normal and abnormal, criminal and innocent, intellectual and mentally retarded, able and disable, etc.

Psychological test provides standardized information about the abilities, capabilities, aptitude, and traits of a person which help in understanding one's personality planning future perspective.

An effectiveness of a particular program is assessed by the application of some kind of test. This function is usually performed by an achievement test. Some experts use tests for research purpose which provide information about the mental level and personality of the subject.

A closely related application of psychological testing is to be found in the selection and classification of military personal.

Industry and business tests are helpful in selection and classifying personal for placement in jobs that range from the simpler semi-skilled, from the selection of filling clerks, sales person to top management of any of these positions. In clinical or mental hospitals, psychological tests are used primarily for individual diagnoses of factors associated with personal problems of learning, behavior attitudes, or specific interpersonal relations.

Personality tests, like other tests used in employee selection, have been under attack for several decades. Personality tests may be seen as an invasion of privacy. Personality tests can be justified if they are able to be used in combination with cognitive ability tests.

In the APA Study in 1997, the American Psychological Association (APA) conducted a study to assess the career outcomes of graduates of accredited university professional psychology programs.

FORENSIC PSYCHOLOGY AND LEGAL SYSTEM

Bartol and Bartol (2008) define forensic psychology as the use of psychology by the legal system. Finally, Bartol and Bartol (2008) reported that the use of psychometric testing has long been a very important part of forensic psychology.

Recently, Gujarat Forensic Sciences University (GFSU) in Gandhinagar, Gujarat (India), started a post-graduation course (Year 2009).

Testing intelligence: Intelligence is distinct from book-learning or test-taking. It was psychologist Alfred Binet who developed the first IQ test to assess students who needed educational assistance. Binet and Theodore Simon developed a set of questions that focused on things not taught in school, including attention, memory, and problem-solving skills.

ROLE OF A NURSE IN PSYCHOLOGICAL ASSESSMENT

Nurse has major role in assessment of psychology. The nurse uses her psychological knowledge in testing the abilities and personality of patients in diagnosis and treatment.

Interests and aptitude tests are very useful in rehabilitation process of a patient. She can decide suitable recreational and occupational training for that patient.

The nurses who go for higher studies and research in psychology definitely need this knowledge. In this way, nurses have a major role **(Fig. 8.3)** to play in psychological assessment.

Components of a Nursing Assessment

In the same way when a report of intelligence test is presented, she should be in a position to know the level of mental retardation in a mentally challenged **(Fig. 8.3)** child. In reporting a neurotic case, she is capable to understand the position and nature of the disease on particular

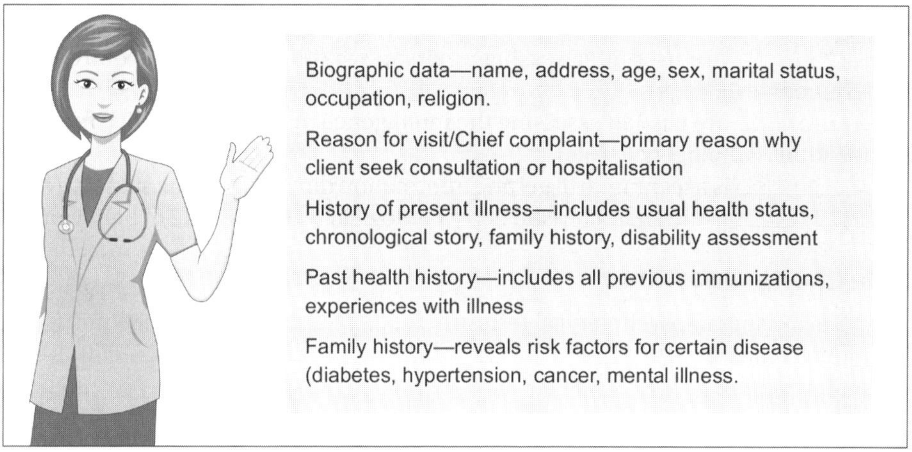

Fig. 8.3: Role of a nurse in psychological assessment

patient. For example, Eysenck Personality Inventory (EPI) is administered to know the level of neuroticism, extraversion, and introversion. Similarly, MMPI is used to know psychoticism and other mental problems.

CONCLUSION

Assessment of psychological conditions of patients is important for intervention in nursing profession. It is very important for the nurse to know what a psychological test is, how tests are constructed and used, what the uses of these tests are, how to interpret the results of tests, etc. The nurse is able to choose an appropriate test to suit particular purpose and particular person. A nurse who has skilled knowledge of psychological assessment can work with team members by building rapport with public. She may plan the tests according to the circumstances. When a report of psychological testing is presented to a nurse, she must be in a position to understand and interpret these results. For example, when an "X-ray" along with report is presented to a nurse, she can definitely understand where the fracture is, what type of fracture, and what precautions must be taken, etc.

QUESTIONS

Essay Question

1. Discuss the types, principles, uses, and nurse's roles in psychological assessment test.

Short Notes

1. Development of psychological tests.
2. Role of nurse in psychological assessment.

Brief Questions

1. Enumerate different psychological assessment tests.
2. Uses of psychological tests.
3. Principles of psychological tests.

Fill in the Blanks

1. ________________ are used in assessing a person what he achieved, acquired or learnt. (Achievement tests)
2. ________________ are used in assessing the intelligence or level of cognitive functioning of the individual. (Intelligence tests)
3. ________________ is a technique of getting information directly from the subject. (Interview)
4. ________________ is the characteristic of psychological tests. (Sample of behavior)

Multiple Choice Questions

1. The characteristics of psychological tests are ....
   a. Sample behavior
   b. Standardisation
   c. Both
2. Development of psychological testing is ....
   a. Intelligence assessment
   b. Guidance
   c. None
3. .... tests are written, verbal evaluation to assess the cognitive emotional functions.
   a. Career planning
   b. Psychological
   c. None

Answers

1. c	2. a	3. b

CHAPTER 9

Application of Soft Skill

Learning Objectives

- Concept of soft skill
- Types of soft skill—visual, aural, and communication skills
- Way of communication
- Building relationship with client and society
- Interpersonal relationships (IPRs)
- Definition, types and purposes, interpersonal skills, and barriers and strategies to overcome barriers
- Survival strategies—managing time, coping stress resilience, and work-life balance
- Applying soft skill to workplace and society
- Use of soft skill in nursing.

CONCEPT OF SOFT SKILL

Soft skill is a professional skill. The term implies to know the personality and attitude of the candidate toward work.

Soft skill is "people's abilities to communicate with each other and work well together".

It is of more importance in company's decision-making in recruitment (According to Cambridge Business English Dictionary).

The Collins English Dictionary defines the term "soft skills" as desirable qualities for certain forms of employment that do not depend on acquired knowledge and they include common sense, the ability to deal with people, and a positive flexible attitude.

A soft skill is a personal attribute of awareness on current situation. It shows the ability of the individual on particular aspect. Soft skills will help the person in job recruitment. It is an emotional intelligence.

In 2018, LinkedIn listed leadership, communication, collaboration, and time management that are most important soft skills.

Soft skills are generally defined as the areas of communication, professionalism, informatics and technology, and leadership and management **(Fig. 9.1)**.

Major companies believe that the person who has high levels of emotional intelligence is good in communication skills, interpersonal skills, and able to achieve goals with team support.

In personal development and communication, train people to express about constructive ways of soft skills to get positive results. Soft skills are generally defined as the areas of communication, professionalism, informatics and technology, and leadership and management.

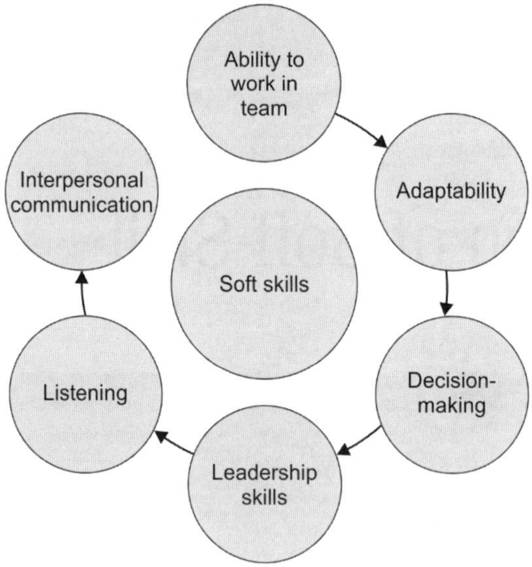

Fig. 9.1: Soft skills

The nurses have to maintain good relationship in work coordination with team support. It helps for successful in treatment. They have to maintain case study, reporting, and medical recording and other technologies. These are possible by development of soft skills in their education process.

TYPES OF SOFT SKILL—VISUAL, AURAL, AND COMMUNICATION SKILLS

Communication is an art of living. It has verbal and nonverbal communication. Verbal communication is the ability of speaking in clarity of information. Nonverbal communication refers with sign, symbol, facial expressions, and body language.

Visual communication is an ability of relay information by using pictures and other visual aids. Visual communication skills require the use of visual aids; eye contact of an individual can also help in visual communication which are read or viewed for ideas and information to be communicated.

Aldous Huxley—Visual communication is regarded as one of the most prominent explores of visual communication and sight-related theories.

Max Wertheimer is father of Gestalt psychology. Gestalt means form of shape in German. In study of Gestalt psychology explains that in principles of perceptual organization visualized shape, continuity and proximity include closure and figure-ground images. These are process of visual communication.

Visual communication in part or whole relies on eyesight. It is included as signs, topography, drawing, graphic design, illustration, industrial design, advertising, animation, color, and electronic resources.

In visual communication, verbal communication is more effective and meaningful by using visual tools and techniques, graphs, or pictures. The television advertisements are motivating the public toward the progress of sales and social awareness on several aspects.

The evaluation of visual communication is based on measurement of comprehension by audience. It refers to the actual presentation of information through a visible medium of text or images.

In study of visual communication, study the basic physics of light, anatomy and physiology of the eye, cognitive and perception theories, color theories, Gestalt psychology, esthetics, design principles, camera/filming actions, and image types, etc. Different professional courses have preferences in approach of practice of these.

Visual aids can play a large role according to the mindset of audience in receiving information by presentation.

Elements in Visual Communication

Objects

It is communication through means that can be read. The use of objects as visual aids helps to bring reality.

Models

The exhibiting-related modes with qualitative and quantitative measures in clarity of information. Examples are human skeletal system, solar system, etc.

Graphs

Graphs are used to differentiate the relationship for clear understanding of messages, line graphs, pie graphs, etc.

Maps

Maps guide the areas to locate destination, distance, etc.

Tables

Tables are columns and rows that organize words, symbols, or data.

Photographs are good tools to recognize for information.

Posters or banners help in visualizing on specific information.

Video is more useful to impress people in publicity. PowerPoint presentation and projectors are very useful in visualizing for educational and motivation programs.

Social media is one of the most effective ways of communication. Text messages and images pass to public by social media.

The mapping, books, posters, design, screen-based media, etc. are more useful visual communication in development of business. Visual communication is becoming an important part of our personal lives as well as professional.

Aural communication is the ability to listen from others saying **(Fig. 9.2)**. Written communication refers as skill in composing text messages, reports, and other types of documents.

"Aural" language, of course, refers to language as we hear it. "Oral" language is what we say. These two words are "homophones"—words spelled differently that sound alike (Author: Peter McKenzie-Brown).

Nurses need soft skills for effective communication in their health profession. They will communicate safer, simple, and qualitative process.

The term "aural" refers to hearing. Aural communication refers to passing along information using the auditory-sensory system using both speaking and hearing.

Oral means to do with the mouth. Aural means to do with the ears. An aural or oral method of communication is one person speaking with their mouth and another person hearing with their ears.

Difference between aural and oral-aural has to do with the ear and hearing. Oral has to do with the mouth or speaking.

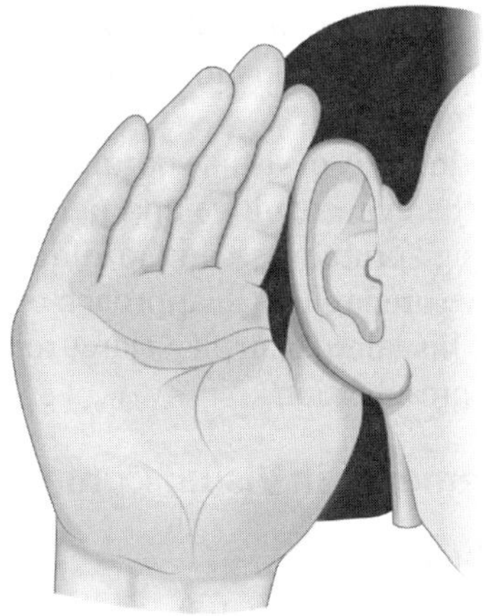

Fig. 9.2: Aural communication method
Source: www.spl-education.blogspot.com

Aural communication can be used to transmit information independently or in combination with visual communication. When conducting surveys, the mode of data collection determines whether information can be transmitted aurally, visually, or both. Whether survey information is transmitted aurally or visually, it influences how respondents first perceive and then cognitively process information to provide their responses.

Aural communication relies heavily on verbal language when information is transmitted through spoken words. Additionally, paralinguistic or paraverbal communication, in which information is conveyed through the speaker's voice, is also an important part of aural communication. Paralinguistic communication can convey additional information.

Aural communication involves in transmitting of information through auditory sense organ. It is the system of speaking and hearing. It is both verbal and nonverbal communication.

Communication of aural used sign, language, Braille, audio, and multimedia by using technology.

WAY OF COMMUNICATION

Communication is a connection among people of society, their thoughts, feelings, ideas, and mutual understanding. Communication refers to the giving and receiving of information. Communication influences behavior and leads to success of nursing interventions. The elements in communication process the sender, message, listener, etc. Communication is both an express opinion to others. The message receiver gives feedback after receiving of message either verbal or nonverbal.

The communication skills are essential for social interactions. The interpersonal communications skills are made to use in business, personal expectations, and priorities in competitive world. In conflict resolutions, effective interpersonal skills are more helpful in both personal and professional life.

BUILDING RELATIONSHIP WITH CLIENT AND SOCIETY

There are three tiers communicational approaches that are desired for interpersonal communicational skills.

1. Strong work for ethic-ethical values—ethics is essential in management of interpersonal relationship among the people and society. Ethics is associated with sentiments and beliefs on different aspects of social environments.
2. Empathy—empathy as one of the important interpersonal skill stands for feelings and thoughts of understanding others in miserable condition of patient or client.
3. Logical—in interpersonal relation, managing logical or analytical way in presentation of views on particular aspect to give clarity in feelings of an individual or group.

Interpersonal skills are vital. These are more efficient even in nonverbal communication of postures, voice, gestures, and eye contact that will express the opinion or interest and sincerity toward others.

INTERPERSONAL SKILL (INTERPERSONAL RELATIONSHIP)

Interpersonal skills are sometimes referred to as social skills or soft skills. In interpersonal skill, it is an ability of communication such as listening, speaking, and control of emotions.

Definition—"the ability to communicate or interact well with other people".

1. Identification of the areas to improve or development
2. Focus on basic communication skill
3. Implement more advanced communications skills to create confidence to listeners.

People with good interpersonal skills are able to work efficiently both at home and office and manages formal and informal groups.

BARRIERS AND STRATEGIES TO OVERCOME BARRIERS

Listening

The listening is also of interpersonal skills. The incomplete theme is not possible to get good answer to the problem solution. Hearing needs patience for completion of process for decision-making.

Teamwork

Teamwork is very useful in achieving desired results in destination. It helps for quick process of decision making, creativity, suggestions by team support.

Problem solving—the person eligible solves complicated problems in critical situations be decision-making.

Decision-making—it is also one of the interpersonal skills in update information for good decision-making by cooperation of team and management.

In organizations, the leader motivates the workers in building team and resolve conflicts to positive atmosphere among the group members. It helps for progress of work and creativity of new ideas in organization.

The interpersonal skills are used daily in communication or interactions with people that is more effective.

SURVIVAL STRATEGIES—MANAGING TIME

Strategic planning is an important skill for employment. In management of consultancy, development of business and analysis of strategic plans have their prominence for survival.

Soft Skills or Survival Skills

The soft skills are survival skills. People use these skills in workplace to avoid distress. These are helping as tools to cope up in employment, business, etc.

The WHO defined burnout as a syndrome caused by "chronic workplace stress that is not successful managed". These skills also help in managing chronic stress in several aspects in teamwork.

Leadership is one of the important soft skills. Leadership needs experience in managing the qualities among the leader in coordination of team and helps in progress of an organization. Most people want to belong to a group and enjoy doing and satisfying to be under good leadership of the organization. It is possible by ability or emotional intelligence of the team leader. The leader exercises authority over authority is willingness and acceptance of the followers. Leader understands the feelings and problems of his followers of his or her team. The leader accepts the responsibility for the actions of the followers without partiality. The leader acquired the qualities to manage the team toward success of his leadership.

Coping Stress Resilience and Work-life Balance

In positive, psychological concept is resilience. It is a sort of miracle drug to heal the sociopsychological traumatic incidents or stressful events in life. It is a wonderful trait to outcome of disappointment or failures.

Modern psychologists describing "resilience is that ineffable quality that allows some people to be knocked down by life and come back stronger than ever. Rather than letting failure overcome them and drain their resolve, they find a way to rise from the ashes".

Resilience is the process of being able to adapt well and bounce back quickly in times of stress. It influences on family, social relations, workplaces, and financial crisis. Developing resilience helps for social adaptation of changes, challenges, etc.

The APA expressed number of factors to contribute and act as markers of resilience.

Capability to make realistic plan and take steps to carry out

Create positive thought and confidence on strength and abilities

Good communication skills and problem solving

Capacity to manage strong feelings and impulses.

APPLYING SOFT SKILLS IN WORKPLACE

Soft skills are useful in workplaces for effective communication, good teamwork, and critical analysis of thoughts for best result. These are useful good initiation of responsible for good administration, leadership to manage quality, and quantity of work for future plans in workplaces. They are also useful in conducting of interviews job recruitment process to assess the ability of skills for development of organization.

The successful of goal and improve the confidence in competing the teams by new adaptation skills in organization.

Goals to Achieve Success in Workplace

- Improvement of communication skills
- Strengthening of teamwork
- Encourage critical and creative thinking.

USE OF SOFT SKILLS IN NURSING

Nursing professionals got the belief on highest levels of honesty and ethical behavior.

Nurses have the responsibility in conveying information, guidance, and advice on physical emotional abilities. The network on health of the patients, doctors, and nurses needs efforts in diagnosis and treatment.

The soft skills can be useful in study of nursing in modification of behavior as psychotherapy skill. In clinical work, supervision using role-play techniques to think alternatives, to differentiate between appropriate and inappropriate, to visualize, and to regulate one's own emotions. Apart from the soft skills required sincerity, genuineness, and openness, it needs at clinical skills in nursing education.

The patient's hope on nurse in availing new health schemes, duration of stay in hospital, and in low budget. It is very difficult to nurse in satisfying the patient in all levels of health progress. It also depends on skills of nurse in communication. It is a challenge to continue developing and fostering professional and interpersonal or "soft skills" among nurses.

Soft skill is a combination of social skill and personality traits. These are more helpful in workplaces with good performance of a competitive world.

The value of skills to student nurse such as communication and leadership in their profession.

According to recent survey, the necessity to learn soft skills for nurse practitioners, nurse administrators, and caretakers of impatient.

CONCLUSION

The student nurse benefits in motivating patient for treatment and help her with coping skills. The efficiency of communication made her in diagnosis by managing health team for quick recovery of illness. In workplaces, the soft skill inspires the employees toward progress of work by resolving conflicts among the team members.

QUESTIONS

Essay Questions

1. What is the concept of soft skill? Explain its importance of communication and interpersonal relation.
2. Explain the importance of strategies of soft skills and uses in nursing profession.

Short Notes

1. Coping stress resilience of soft skill.
2. How soft skills are strategies to overcome barriers?

Brief Questions

1. What do you mean by soft skill?
2. Define resilience.

Fill in the Blanks

1. Communication, teamwork, and listening are ________________ skills. (soft)
2. In interpersonal ________________, it is an ability of communication such as listening, speaking, and control of emotions. (skill)

Multiple Choice Questions

1. Communication, team work is .... skill.
   a. Dramatic
   b. Soft
   c. Both
2. Soft skill is a combination of social .... and personality traits.
   a. Skill
   b. Trait
   c. Both

Answers

1. b	2. a

CHAPTER 10

Self-empowerment

Learning Objectives

- Self-empowerment
- Dimensions of self-empowerment
- Self-empowerment and development
- Importance of women's empowerment on society
- Professional etiquette in personal grooming
- Role of nurse in empowering others.

INTRODUCTION

Empowerment is a set of measures designed to increase the degree of autonomy and self-determination. It represents their interests in a responsible and self-determined way, acting on their own authority.

Empowerment is well-researched areas in nursing practice in terms of culture and socialization. The student nurse learns all these in practice of social interactions to educate patients and communities. She uses empowerment in teamwork and power to reach goal.

Self-empowerment means taking caring of their own life. The base of self-empowerment is peace. Self-empowerment helps in transition of person's disappointment and frustration to lead peaceful life.

Self-empowerment states that the first word self means own thoughts, desires, and individuality. The major thought of self not to convince the mind even in storm situations. Empowerment means power or capacity to exercise control or authority and the ability to accomplish guide.

DIMENSIONS IN SELF-EMPOWERMENT

The term empowerment has long interesting history in social movements, struggle for justice, and to gain equalities in conflicts. In modern society, it is more useful in self-improvement, individualism, etc.

PLANNING IN DECISION-MAKING

In self-empowerment focuses on control of policies in decision-making, self-determination and authoritative power are essential in some aspects of both personal and professional life. The decision has to be motivational and responsible process in reaching goal.

CREATIVE INPUT

The created ideas have special status in developmental process of decision-making. It is more effective in organizational process to cope up in working areas to manage teamwork.

SOURCES FOR NOVELTY

The sources search is essential in specific subject for initiation of improving of new skills. The role of team members and their skills has to be effective for acceptance and contribution in organization. It depends on their communication and empowerment in group activities. The administrative strategies help for development of strategies linked with empowerment.

SUPPORT OF WORKING GROUP

The support of employees is very important in development of organization. The role of every employee in all levels from lower to higher has major role in implementation of all these in working areas. The investigation and researches on new policies in plan of development were possible by empowerment of employees in organization. The influence of all these improve the value and competitive spirit in business organization.

GROUP DECISION-MAKING

The importance of group member ideas is valuable in assessment, changing policies by evaluation, and verification process in decision-making done by the support of all categories for final determination of goal. This is more powerful concept for new employees in motivational process for work progress in organizational future.

IMPORTANCE OF WOMEN'S EMPOWERMENT ON SOCIETY

In societal empowerment of women, it is based on three basics—personal, relational, and societal aspects. The gender discrimination is also giving prominence in women empowerment in leading life in society. It is more essential for women to get financial support and in eradication of poverty with women empowerment and taking role in earning.

The illiteracy, poverty, and superstitions are challenging by self-empowerment in women of Indian society. Empowerment helps in increasing living standards of human life. The joint family system is decreased, migration to cities, and scarcity of resources also creating social awareness for empowerment.

The self-empowerment through education inspires women to use in daily life. It leads for comfortable life and progress of society. Self-empowerment is essential for every woman of Indian society. It helps in all aspects of their growth in both personal and professional life. It is more useful for not only career development and also for social interaction.

Self is a state of all powerful love, truth effects to deal challenges, and struggle to gain ability in achievement of lovable things.

Women's empowerment is an important goal in achievement of success. There are three dimensions:

1. Individual personal beliefs as well as actions are to be observed
2. Relation to these beliefs and actions to be observed in empowerment
3. The outcome of societal context where societal empowerment can also be observed.

In society cultural aspects, its influence on women's empowerment and the gap between cultural changes between material and nonmaterial culture affect the dimensions in intervention of empowerment. Women empowerment improves ability in understanding the results of comparison in several aspects of social environment developing strategies, designing, planning, and interpretation. In this process, the usage of resources and agencies is considered to be basics in women empowerment. Indian society is male dominant society. The women faced struggle for achievement to equal role in self-determination and success.

Psychological stress is sensitive in tolerating cultural aspects of orthodox families and beliefs as barrier in empowerment of women. Most of the psychological researches on women empowerment are thought of moral and ethical values for the well-being of the family and social environment.

The satisfying sense of harmony on women's empowerment emerges from various sources of society. Empowering women is good in positive attitude in societal relations of families, children, and communities. It helps to reduce poverty and psychological and income generation.

PROFESSIONAL ETIQUETTE IN PERSONAL GROOMING

Etiquette is the customary code of polite behavior in society or among members of particular profession in group.

British English defines "Etiquette is a set of customs and rules for polite behavior, especially among a particular class of people or in a particular profession".

Etiquette is a conventional but unwritten code of practice followed by members of any of certain professions or groups in medical etiquette.

In American English, etiquette means 'the forms, manners, and ceremonies established by conventions as acceptable or required in social relations, in a profession or in social life".

Etiquette training is a key point of soft skills and communication for acceptance behavior in professional process.

In development of professional companies focusing attention on cultural aspects, communication in usage of mobile phones and international protocols are in training etiquette. Etiquette training is an important program.

Professional etiquette focuses on:

1. Enhancement of social skills
2. Confidential interaction
3. Ability of positive attitude
4. Ability to improve good verbal and nonverbal communication skills
5. Ability to improve good conversational ability by phone
6. Ability to interact in meeting or conference with soft skills.

Greater awareness of grooming and etiquette skills will help to create confidence in formal, professional, and social situations.

Body language is also one of the important topics in professional etiquette. It creates positive impression in understanding language and vocabulary to impress others toward success of goal.

In lifestyle dressing, it is also important to manage color contrast, dignity in executives, authoritative, in policy implementation, and associated with moral values and ethics in professional circle to manage teamwork in workplaces. Punctuality and sincerity create confidence in professional aspect among the teamwork by empowerment.

Professionals need to understand that grooming themselves to build personality, confidence, and ability to impress among colleagues. The professional behavior clearly appears in their walking style, speech, dressing, hairstyle, and mannerism in social interactions and organizational settings.

The professional etiquette in women has great importance in personality traits; approach with other team members creates confidence to opposite gender with ethical values, respect, and safety in team participation of workplaces. Especially choice of dress color, model of dress, and neatness are very important in managing professional etiquette in personal grooming.

ROLE OF NURSING IN EMPOWERING OTHER

Empowerment is more important in nursing profession. The proper training is essential for every nurses in social interaction in all areas of health. It helps for warning sign in motivation for good health and prevention of illness.

CONCLUSION

Power is widely used concept in both physical and social sciences. It is an energy to prove efficiency or skill to get progress and development of every activity. The empowerment has great importance in both psychological and physical activities in improvement of personal traits. Nursing is more essential for both personal and professional life.

QUESTIONS

Essay Questions

1. Describe meaning of self-empowerment. As a nurse, how can you apply this in your profession?
2. Explain as a woman the uses of self-empowerment in society.

Short Questions

1. What are the dimensions of self-empowerment?
2. Define the role of nurse in empowering others.

Brief Question

1. What is "Professional etiquette"?

Fill in the Blanks

1. ________________ means power or capacity to exercise control or authority and the ability to accomplish guide. (Empowerment)
2. ________________ is the customary code of polite behavior in society or among members of particular profession in group. (Etiquette)

Multiple Choice Questions

1. .... means power or capacity to exercise control or authority and the ability to accomplish guide.
   a. Empowerment
   b. Etiquette
   c. Both
2. In choice of dress color, model of dress, neatness is very important in managing professional .... in personal grooming.
   a. Empowerment
   b. Etiquette
   c. Both

Answers

1. a	2. b

Previous University Examination Papers

NTR University of Health Sciences, Vijayawada, Andhra Pradesh
BSc (Nursing) Degree Examinations—November, 2015
First year Examination—4 YDC
Psychology (New Scheme)

Time: 3 Hours **Marks: 75**

Answer the following questions

1. **Write an essay on any TWO of the following:** **15 × 2 = 30**
   a. Define intelligence. Explain theories of intelligence
   b. Discuss the types, principles, uses and nurse's role in psychological assessment test.
   c. Explain the types, development and theories of memory.
2. **Write short notes on any FIVE of the following:** **5 × 5 = 25**
   a. Describe coping during stress.
   b. Define personality and discuss any one type.
   c. Relevance of psychology in nursing.
   d. Explain psychology of sensation.
   e. Enumerate defence mechanisms and explain any three.
   f Concept of mental hygiene.
   g. Explain behavior and attitude.
3. **Write brief answers of the following:** **10 × 2 = 20**
   a Define learner and learning.
   b. Meaning about guidance and counseling.
   c. Definition of psychology and its methods.
   d. Enumerate types of hallucination.
   e. Write the aptitude in individual difference.
   f. List down the cognitive process of psychometric assessment.
   g. Difine conflict.
   h. Define the duration and degree of attention.
   i. Define genetics and behavior.
   j. Lsit down the scope of psychology in nursing

NTR University of Health Sciences, Vijayawada, Andhra Pradesh

BSc (Nursing) Degree Examinations—June, 2016

First year Examination—4 YDC

Psychology—(New Scheme)

Time: 3 Hours **Max. Marks: 75**

Answer the following questions

1. **Write an essay on any TWO of the following:** **2 × 15 = 30 marks**
   a. Explain the effect of heredity and environment on human behavior.
   b. Explain the trait theories of personality. Discuss the various trait compositions necessary to have effective Nurse patient relationship.
   c. Define guidance and counseling. List down the principles of guidance and counseling.
2. **Write short notes on any FIVE of the following:** **5 × 5 = 25**
   a. Experimental method.
   b. Conditioning theories of learning.
   c. Conflict and frustration.
   d. Distribution of intelligence.
   e. Factors that control and divert attention.
   f. Evaluate the theories of emotions.
   g. Endocrine glands and their functions.
3. **Write brief answers on the following:** **10 × 2 = 20**
   a. Write the meaning of introspection.
   b. Define para-psychology.
   c. Name the types of sensory memory.
   d. Define synapse.
   e. Enumerate the different types of thinking.
   f. List the types of amnesia.
   g. Enlist the sources of Stressors.
   h. Define attitude change.
   i. Write the meaning of social motives.
   j. Enumerate the types of developmental psychology.

NTR University of Health Sciences, Vijayawada, Andhra Pradesh

BSc (Nursing) Degree Examinations—November, 2016

First year Examination—4 YDC

Psychology (New Scheme)

Time: 3 Hours **Marks: 75**

Answer the following questions

1. **Write an essay on any TWO of the following:** **2× 15 = 30 marks**
   a. A. Define emotion. B. Explain the theories of emotions. C. Narrate emotions in health and sickness. 2 + 8 + 5 = 15
   b. A. Define personality. B. Explain about psychoanalytic theory of personality.2 + 13 = 15
   c. A. Define psychology. B. Explain its nature and scope with special reference to nursing. 2 + 13 = 15

2. **Write short notes on any FIVE of the following:** **5 × 5 = 25**
   a. Write briefly on warning signs of poor mental health.
   b. Explain trial and error learning.
   c. Illustrate the factors determining perception.
   d. Write in detail about the factors determining perception.
   e. Definition and types of motivation.
   f. Justify the influence of heredity and environment on behavior.
   g. Define thinking and explain the types of thinking.

3. **Write brief answers on the following:** **10 × 2 = 20**
   a. Write the formula for calculating Intelligence Quotient.
   b. Define span of attention.
   c. List the advantages of reinforcement.
   d. Define creative thinking.
   e. Define sensation
   f. Define sublimation
   g. Write the meaning of Amnesia
   h. Define id, ego and superego.
   j. Enumerate the types of conflicts
   i. Mention any four physical traits.

NTR University of Health Sciences, Vijayawada, Andhra Pradesh

BSc (Nursing) Degree Examinations—June, 2017

First year Examination—4 YDC

Psychology (New Scheme)

Time: 3 Hours **Max. Marks: 75**

1. **Write an essay on any TWO of the following:** **2 × 15 = 30 marks**
   a. Define psychology and critically discuss the merits and demerits of the different methods used in the study of psychology.
   b. Define intelligence. Explain the assessment of intelligence and write the applications of intelligence.
   c. Explain heredity and environment and their effect in human behavior.
2. **Write short notes on any FIVE of the following:** **5 × 5 = 25**
   a. Stress and coping
   b. Effect of reward and punishment on learning.
   c. Discuss the stages of development in thinking.
   d. Factors influencing the level of attention.
   e. Guidance and counseling.
   f. Different types of memory.
   g. Characteristics of mentally healthy person.
3. **Write brief answers on the following:** **10 × 2 = 20**
   a. Write the differences between illusion and hallucination
   b. Enlist the types of attitude.
   c. Define extra sensory perception.
   d. Write the differences between eustress and distress
   e. Name the laws of learning.
   f. Distinguish between the extravert and introvert.
   g. Define personal motives.
   h. Enumerate Endocrine glands.
   i. Name the parts of neuron.
   j. List out four types of defence mechanisms.

NTR University of Health Sciences, Vijayawada, Andhra Pradesh

BSc (Nursing) Degree Examinations—November, 2017

First year Examination—4 YDC

Psychology (New Scheme)

Time: 3 Hours **Max. Marks: 75**

1. **Write an essay on any TWO of the following:** **2 × 15 = 30 marks**
   a. Define intelligence and write application in detail.
   b. Explain the assessment of intelligence and write application in detail.
   c. Discuss the types, determinants and alteration of attention.
   d. Explain types, theories of motivation and narrate conflict resolution.
2. **Write short notes on any FIVE of the following:** **5 × 5 = 25**
   a. List down the principles of counseling.
   b. Write any one learning theory.
   c. Illustrate the factors affecting behavior and attitudes.
   d. Describe the errors in perception.
   e. How does the thinking influence the language and communication.
   g. Explain the methods of memorising and describe forgetting.
   h. Explain the promotive mental health strategies and services
3. **Write brief answers on the following:** **10 × 2 = 20**
   a. List the types of personality.
   b. Define guidance.
   c. Mention any two effects of stressors.
   d. Write the nature and behavior of organism.
   e. Define health and illness.
   f. List the silent features of topography of personality.
   g. Mention the components emotions.
   h. List any four features of psychology of sick people.
   i. Difference between ego and superego.
   j. Define study habits.

NTR University of Health Sciences, Vijayawada, Andhra Pradesh

BSc (Nursing) Degree Examinations—June, 2018

First year Examination—4 YDC

Psychology (New Scheme)

Time: 3 Hours **Max. Marks: 75**

1. **Write an essay on any TWO of the following:** **2 × 15 = 30 marks**
   a. Define attitude. B. Explain factors involved in attitude change. C. Write in detail about psychometric assessment of attitude. 2 + 7 + 6 = 15
   b. A. Define learning. B. Explain the types of learning. C. Explain the theories of learning. 2 + 4+ 9 = 15
   c. A. State heredity and environment. B. Give an account of the role of heredity and environment in causing individual difference. C. Narrate the significance of psychology in nursing. 3 + 7 + 5 = 15
2. **Write short notes on any FIVE of the following:** **5 × 5 = 25**
   a. Differentiate between illusion and hallucination with examples.
   b. Explain source of stress.
   c. Explain types and process of thinking.
   d. Types of conflict and methods to solve it.
   e. Brief about grief and stages.
   f. Enlist the defence mechanisms and explain any three in detail.
   g. Detail the methods of memorising.
3. **Write brief answers on the following:** **10 × 2 = 20**
   a. Differentiate between Emotions and feelings.
   b. Differentiate between projection and rationalisation.
   c. Differentiate between mental age and chronological age
   d. Differentiate between incentives and reinforcement.
   e. Define transfer of learning.
   f. Define experimental psychology.
   g. Define extrovert.
   h. Define biological motive.
   i. Define integrated response.
   j. Differentiate between aptitude and attitude.

NTR University of Health Sciences, Vijayawada, Andhra Pradesh

BSc (Nursing) Degree Examinations—November, 2018

First year Examination—4 YDC

Psychology (New Scheme)

Time: 3 Hours **Max. Marks: 75**

1. **Write an essay on any TWO of the following:** **2 × 15 = 30 marks**
   a. Define stress. List the stressors and explain adaptation and coping.
   b. A. Define perception. Discuss the principle of perception. B. Explain the errors in perception.
   c. Define psychology. Why is psychology necessary for nursing? B. Explain the methods of psychology.
   d. Explain types, theories of motivation and narrate conflict resolution.
2. **Write short notes on any FIVE of the following:** **5 × 5 = 25**
   a. Describe the psychology of sensation.
   b. Explain the psychology of adolescence.
   c. Describe the relation between language and communication.
   d. Enlist the ego defence mechanisms—explain any one.
   e. Explain types of attitudes.
   f. Characteristics of mentally healthy person.
   g. Assessment of personality.
3. **Write brief answers on the following:** **10 × 2 = 20**
   a. Define study habits.
   b. List the process of guidance.
   c. Enumerate the psychology of women.
   d. Define the determinants of attention.
   e. Define conflict and frustration.
   f. Define amnesia.
   g. Enumerate the classification of intelligence.
   h. Mention any two features of variability in attitude.
   i. List the types of personality.
   j. List the salient features of motives and behavior.

NTR University of Health Sciences, Vijayawada, Andhra Pradesh

BSc (Nursing) Degree Examinations—June, 2019

First year Examination—4 YDC

Psychology (New Scheme)

Time: 3 Hours **Max. Marks: 75**

1. **Write an essay on any TWO of the following:** **2 × 15 = 30 marks**
   a. Define emotions. List its components and narrate emotions in health and illness.
   b. Define personality. Write the types and the psychometric assessments of personality.
   c. Discuss meaning, principles and factors affecting perception.

2. **Write short notes on any FIVE of the following:** **5 × 5 = 25**
   a. Explain the theories and methods of memorising.
   b. Narrate the process of counseling.
   c. Describe the classification of intelligence.
   d. How does heredity and environment influences the behavior.
   e. Explain the attitudinal change.
   f. Describe the importance of psychology in nursing.
   g. Explain the process of body mind relationship with health and illness.

3. **Write brief answers on the following:** **10 × 2 = 20**
   a. Define mental hygiene.
   b. Enumerate the strategies of preventive mental health.
   c. Explain the duration and degree of attention.
   d. Define brain and behavior.
   e. Difference between ego and Superego.
   f. Explain stress cycle.
   g. List any two influences of study habits in learning.
   h. Define psychology of sensation.
   i. Define aptitude.
   j. Enumerate the types of thinking.

NTR University of Health Sciences, Vijayawada, Andhra Pradesh

BSc (Nursing) Degree Examinations—November, 2019

First year Examination—4 YDC

Psychology (New Scheme)

Time: 3 Hours **Max. Marks: 75**

1. **Write an essay on any TWO of the following:** **2 × 15 = 30 marks**
   a. How would you define thinking? Enlist types of thinking? Explain its relationship with language and communication.
   b. Define motivation and reinforcement. Explain Maslow's hierarchy of needs and draw details about social motives.
   c. Define intelligence. Explain theories of intelligence.
2. **Write short notes on any FIVE of the following:** **5 × 5 = 25**
   a. Write any one learning theory.
   b. Explain the causes of individual differences.
   c. Describe emotions that encourage health and facts that hamper the healthy functioning of the body.
   d. Describe coping during stress.
   e. Enumerate defence mechanisms and explain any three of them.
   f. Briefly describe organisation of personality.
   g. Characteristics of mentally healthy person.
3. **Write brief answers on the following:** **10 × 2 = 20**
   a. Define abstract thinking.
   b. Define genes.
   c. Difference between regression and suppression.
   d. Difference between illusion and hallucination
   e. Difference between ego and Superego.
   f. Formula for calculating intelligence quotient.
   g. Define superego.
   h. Enumerate importance of psychology in nursing.
   i. Define division of attention.
   j. Enlist the advantages of projective test.

Index

Page numbers followed by *f* refer to figure, and *t* refer to table

S

T

V

W